Milady's Nail Technology Workbook

Second Edition

STUDENT'S EDITION

Online Services

Delmar Online
To access a wide variety of Delmar products and services on the World Wide Web, point your browser to:
   http://www.delmar.com/delmar.html
   or email: info@delmar.com

thomson.com
To access International Thomson Publishing's home site for information on more than 34 publishers and 20,000 products, point your browser to:
   http://www.thomson.com
   or email: findit@kiosk.thomson.com

Milady's Nail Technology Workbook

Second Edition

STUDENT'S EDITION

To be used with
MILADY'S ART AND SCIENCE OF NAIL TECHNOLOGY

Compiled by Linnea Lindquist

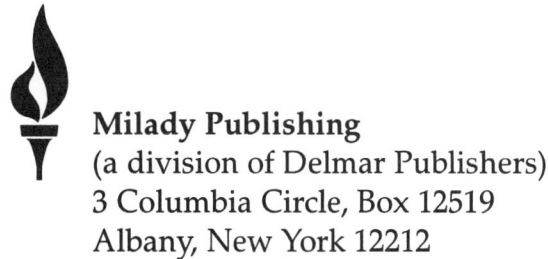

Milady Publishing
(a division of Delmar Publishers)
3 Columbia Circle, Box 12519
Albany, New York 12212

NOTICE TO THE READER

Publisher does not warrant or guarantee any of the products described herein or perform any independent analysis in connection with any of the product information contained herein. Publisher does not assume, and expressly disclaims, any obligation to obtain and include information other than that provided to it by the manufacturer.

The reader is expressly warned to consider and adopt all safety precautions that might be indicated by the activities herein and to avoid all potential hazards. By following the instructions contained herein, the reader willingly assumes all risks in connections with such instructions.

The publisher makes no representation or warranties of any kind, including but not limited to, the warranties of fitness for particular purpose or merchantability, nor are any such representations implied with respect to the material set forth herein, and the publisher takes no responsibility with respect to such material. The publisher shall not be liable for any special, consequential, or exemplary damages resulting, in whole or part, from the readers' use of, or reliance upon, this material.

Photographer: Michael A. Gallitelli, on location at the Austin Beauty School, with Dino Petrocelli

Medical Photographers:
Elvin Zook, MD
Southern Illinois University
School of Medicine
Springfield, IL

Orville J. Stone, MD
Dermatology Medical Group
Huntington Beach, CA

Technical Consultant: Tanya Severino

Artists:
Shizuko Horii
Ron Young

The staff of Milady Publishing Company wishes to thank the following people who contributed to this publication:

Carol Laubach
San Jacinto College
Pasadena, TX

Laura Manicho
Nationwide Beauty Academy
Cols, OH

Marion McWhorter
San Jacinto College
Pasadena, TX

Sandra Skoney
Toledo Academy of Beauty Culture
Toledo, OH

Linda Zizzo
Milwaukee Area Technical College
Milwaukee, WI

COPYRIGHT © 1997
Milady Publishing
(a division of Delmar Publishers)

an International Thomson Publishing company I(T)P®

Printed in the United States of America

For more information, contact:
Milady Publishing
3 Columbia Circle, Box 12519
Albany, New York 12212-2519

All rights reserved. No part of this work covered by the copyright hereon may be reproduced or used in any form or by any means—graphic, electronic, or mechanical, including photocopying, recording, taping, or information storage and retrieval systems—without the written permission of the publisher.

ISBN: 1-56253-327-4

Library of Congress Catalog Number: 96-35281

10 9 8 7 6 5 4 3

Contents

How to Use This Workbook vii
Introduction 1

PART 1: GETTING STARTED   3
1 Your Professional Image 4
2 Bacteria and Other Infectious Agents 8
3 Sanitation and Disinfection 15
4 Safety in the Salon 19

PART 2: THE SCIENCE OF NAIL TECHNOLOGY   25
5 Nail Product Chemistry Simplified 26
6 Anatomy and Physiology 29
7 The Nail and Its Disorders 43
8 The Skin and Its Disorders 51
9 Client Consultation 59

PART 3: BASIC PROCEDURES   61
10 Manicuring 62
11 Pedicuring 73

PART 4: THE ART OF NAIL TECHNOLOGY   79
12 Nail Tips 80
13 Nail Wraps 85
14 Acrylic Nails 91
15 Gels 100
16 The Creative Touch 105

PART 5: THE BUSINESS OF NAIL TECHNOLOGY   109
17 Salon Business 110
18 Selling Nail Products and Services 115
    Final Review 119

How to Use This Workbook

Milady's Nail Technology Workbook has been written to meet the needs, interests, and abilities of students receiving training in nail technology.

This workbook should be used together with *Milady's Art and Science of Nail Technology*. This book follows the information found in the student textbook.

Students are to answer each item in this workbook with a pencil after consulting their textbook for correct information. Items can be corrected and/or rated during class or individual discussions, or on an independent study basis.

Various tests are included to emphasize essential facts found in the textbook and to measure the student's progress. "Word Reviews" are listed for each chapter. They are to be used as study guides, for class discussions, or for the teacher to assign groups of words to be used by the student in creative essays.

Date _____

Rating _____

Text Pages 1-4

Introduction

1. List four advantages of becoming a nail technician in today's cosmetology profession.
   a. _____
   b. _____
   c. _____
   d. _____

2. This booming industry includes manicuring, _____, and _____.

3. The nail industry had a combined sales of more than _____ per year, which is an increase of more than _____ over previous years.

4. Besides becoming a nail technician, list five other career opportunities available to you.
   a. _____
   b. _____
   c. _____
   d. _____
   e. _____

5. The first manicure was recorded _____ years ago.

6. Discuss items nail technicians learn while in training for licensure.
   a. _____
   b. _____
   c. _____
   d. _____
   e. _____
   f. _____

7. a. What does the Latin word "manus" mean?
      _____

   b. What does the Latin word "cura" mean?
      _____

1

Part 1

GETTING STARTED

- ◆ *CHAPTER 1* - Your Professional Image
- ◆ *CHAPTER 2* - Bacteria and Other Infectious Agents
- ◆ *CHAPTER 3* - Sanitation and Disinfection
- ◆ *CHAPTER 4* - Safety in the Salon

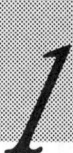

Date _____

Rating _____

Text Pages 6-13

Your Professional Image

INTRODUCTION

1. The three groups of people that will be affected by rules for professional behavior are

   a. _____.
   b. _____.
   c. _____.

2. List three elements that are included in the rules of professionalism.

   a. _____
   b. _____
   c. _____

PROFESSIONAL SALON CONDUCT

3. Define salon conduct.

   _____

   _____

4. List twelve items concerning salon conduct toward clients.

   a. _____
   b. _____
   c. _____
   d. _____
   e. _____
   f. _____
   g. _____
   h. _____
   i. _____
   j. _____
   k. _____
   l. _____

5. Being late is discourteous and can annoy and _____ your clients.

6. What four items should be included on an appointment schedule?

   a. _____

   b. _____

   c. _____

   d. _____

7. Schedule your appointments so that each client has enough _____.

8. a. List two situations when you should contact your clients about schedule changes.

   1. _____

   2. _____

   b. By contacting clients for the above two situations, your clients will

   1. _____

   2. _____

9. List three parts of a courteous attitude.

   a. _____

   b. _____

   c. _____

10. What five actions should be performed for a new client?

    a. _____

    b. _____

    c. _____

    d. _____

    e. _____

11. Explain why a nail technician should not chew gum, smoke, or eat when with a client.
    _____

12. List ten items concerning salon conduct toward employers and coworkers.

    a. _____

    b. _____

    c. _____

    d. _____

    e. _____

    f. _____

    g. _____

    h. _____

    i. _____

    j. _____

13. a. Problems or questions about your job should be discussed with your _____ .
    b. These problems or questions should not be discussed with your
       1. _____
       2. _____

PROFESSIONAL ETHICS

14. Define professional ethics.
    _____
    _____

15. List four essential values when considering the feelings and rights of others.
    a. _____
    b. _____
    c. _____
    d. _____

16. Write down seven professional ethical behaviors toward clients.
    a. _____
    b. _____
    c. _____
    d. _____
    e. _____
    f. _____
    g. _____

17. Explain why a nail technician should not gossip about others to clients.
    _____
    _____

18. List five professional ethical behaviors with employers and coworkers.
    a. _____
    b. _____
    c. _____
    d. _____
    e. _____

YOUR PROFESSIONAL APPEARANCE

19. Give three reasons why you should be a model of good grooming.
    a. _____
    b. _____
    c. _____

20. List four actions of good grooming.

   a. _____
   b. _____
   c. _____
   d. _____

COMPLETION REVIEW

Insert the correct word listed in the sentences below.

appearance	coworkers	professional ethics
appointment schedule	employers	salon conduct
calendar	helpful	time
clients	inconvenience	

21. Being late is discourteous, and can annoy and _____ your clients.

22. The parts of a courteous attitude include being cheerful, friendly, and _____.

23. The way you act when you are working with clients, your employer, and coworkers in a salon is called _____.

24. Schedule your appointments so that each client has enough _____.

25. Problems or questions about your job should be discussed with your _____.

26. Clients expecting you to look your best refers to your professional _____.

27. The client's name and phone number, service, and time should be included on a/an _____.

28. Your sense of right or wrong when you interact with your clients, employers, and coworkers is known as _____.

WORD REVIEW

If you do not know the meanings of the words listed below, look them up in the text.

appearance	efficient	prepare
appointment schedule	employer	professional
argue	ethical standards	promote
communication	ethics	punctual
complain	fairness	respect
courteous	good grooming	rumors
courtesy	gossip	salon conduct
coworkers	honesty	
criticize	initiative	

2

Date _____

Rating _____

Text Pages 14-24

Bacteria and Other Infectious Agents

INTRODUCTION

1. List four sources of infection.

    a. _____
    b. _____
    c. _____
    d. _____

BACTERIA

2. Define bacteria.

   _____

3. List some places where bacteria are found.

    a. _____
    b. _____
    c. _____
    d. _____
    e. _____
    f. _____
    g. _____
    h. _____
    i. _____
    j. _____
    k. _____

4. **Identification.** Using the letters **P** and **NP** (defined below), match the characteristics below with one type of bacteria.

    Key:

    P = pathogenic bacteria

    NP = nonpathogenic bacteria

    Characteristics

    _____ a. less than 30% of all bacteria

    _____ b. are often beneficial

_____ c. spread disease by producing toxins/poisons
_____ d. help produce food and oxygen
_____ e. in the mouth and intestines they help the digestive process
_____ f. non-disease-causing
_____ g. 70% of all bacteria
_____ h. harmful bacteria
_____ i. cocci, bacilli, spirilla
_____ j. most common cause of infection and disease

5. List four conditions in which bacteria live, grow, and multiply.

   a. _____
   b. _____
   c. _____
   d. _____

6. a. Define and explain mitosis.

   _____
   _____
   _____

   b. How many bacteria cells can be reproduced in 12 hours?

   _____

7. a. Define spore.

   _____
   _____

   b. When does this spore form?

   _____
   _____

   c. When will the bacteria grow and reproduce again?

   _____
   _____

8. **Identification.** Using the letters **C, B,** and **S** (defined below), match the characteristics below with one type of pathogenic bacteria.

   Key
   C = cocci bacteria
   B = bacilli bacteria
   S = spirilla bacteria

   Characteristics
   _____ a. the most common bacteria
   _____ b. causes influenza and typhoid
   _____ c. causes strep throat and blood poisoning

9

        _____ d. spiral-shaped

        _____ e. causes local infections, such as boils

        _____ f. includes treponema pallida

        _____ g. rod-shaped

        _____ h. diplococci causes pneumonia

        _____ i. causes syphilis

        _____ j. corkscrew-shaped

        _____ k. round, pus-producing bacteria

        _____ l. causes tuberculosis and diphtheria

9. a. Which two types of bacteria can propel themselves?

    1. _____

    2. _____

  b. The hairlike projections by which they move are called _____ or _____ .

VIRUSES

10. Define viruses.

_____

_____

11. List in order the actions of viruses.

  a. _____

  b. _____

  c. _____

12. Viruses can be transformed through casual contact and spread when a person sneezes or _____ .

13. **Identification**. Using the letters **B** and **V** (defined below), match the diseases below with their cause.

  Key:

  B = bacteria-caused disease

  V = virus-caused disease

Diseases:

  _____ a. pustules   _____ g. rheumatic fever

  _____ b. common cold   _____ h. chicken pox

  _____ c. measles   _____ i. AIDS

  _____ d. tetanus   _____ j. strep throat

  _____ e. mumps

  _____ f. syphilis

14. a. What do the letters AIDS stand for?
    _____

    b. What does the AIDS virus attack and eventually destroy?
    _____

    c. What are two common methods of transferring AIDS?
        1. _____
        2. _____

    d. What should you tell a client who is concerned about the spread of AIDS in the salon?
    _____
    _____

FUNGUS AND MOLD, PARASITES AND RICKETTSIA

15. **Matching.** Match the terms on the left with their correct descriptions on the right.

    _____ 1. fungi
    _____ 2. mold
    _____ 3. rickettsia
    _____ 4. nail fungus
    _____ 5. parasites

    A. rarely, if ever, appears on fingernails; commonly confused with greenish bacterial infection
    B. causes AIDS and blood poisoning
    C. multicelled animal or plant organisms
    D. appears as a discoloration under the nail plate that spreads toward the cuticle
    E. one-celled plant microorganisms
    F. caused when the natural nail and products put on it are sanitized
    G. the general term for plantlike parasites
    H. causes typhus and Rocky Mountain fever

16. a. Should a nail technician perform services on a client who has nail fungus?
    _____

    b. Why or why not?
    _____

17. a. Explain what parasites live off.
    _____

    b. An example of a plant parasite is _____ .

    c. List three examples of animal parasites.
        1. _____
        2. _____
        3. _____

18. Explain safety precautions that should be used when removing an artificial nail covering for a person who has nail fungus or other infection.

    a. _____
    b. _____
    c. _____
       _____
    d. _____
       _____

UNDERSTANDING INFECTION

19. a. Explain when an infection occurs.
       _____
       _____

    b. At first, the infection is _____ .
    c. If the infection spreads to the bloodstream, it is called a _____ infection.

20. **Matching.** Match the terms of the left with their correct descriptions on the right.

    _____ 1. immunity
    _____ 2. artificially acquired immunity
    _____ 3. general infection
    _____ 4. naturally acquired immunity
    _____ 5. localized infection
    _____ 6. natural immunity

    A. broken skin and lack of perspiration/bodily secretions
    B. ability of the body to resist disease and destroy microorganisms when they have entered the body
    C. often the first stage of an infection
    D. injection of serum or vaccine that introduces a small dose of disease-causing microorganisms into the body
    E. attacks and eventually destroys the body's immune system
    F. unbroken skin, natural secretions, and the blood's white blood cells
    G. after fighting off a disease, antibodies remain in the bloodstream
    H. the body's inability to resist disease-causing microorganisms
    I. example is blood poisoning

21. List five ways in which bacteria, viruses, and fungi enter the body.

    a. _____
    b. _____
    c. _____
    d. _____
    e. _____

22. List five common sources of infections for nail technicians.

   a. _____
   b. _____
   c. _____
   d. _____
   e. _____

23. Explain four ways nail technicians can fight infections.

   a. _____
   b. _____
   c. _____
   d. _____

MATCHING REVIEW

Insert the correct word listed in front of each definition below.

acquired immunity	immunity	pediculosis
AIDS	mitosis	ringworm
bacilli	natural immunity	scabies
bacteria	nonpathogenic	spirilla
cocci	parasites	spore
flagella	pathogenic	virus

24. _____ cell division

25. _____ common name for acquired immune deficiency syndrome

26. _____ type of bacteria that causes strep throat and blood poisoning

27. _____ multicelled animal or plant organisms

28. _____ one-celled microorganisms so small they can only be seen through a microscope

29. _____ bacteria move by these hairlike projections

30. _____ disease-causing agents that are many times smaller than bacteria

31. _____ a plant parasite that is contagious

32. _____ harmful bacteria including cocci, spirilla, and bacilli

33. _____ ability of the body to resist disease and destroy microorganisms when they have entered the body

34. _____ a tough outer covering on some bacteria

35. _____ spiral-shaped bacteria that causes syphilis

36. _____ non-disease causing, may be beneficial

37. _____ includes unbroken skin, natural secretions, and the blood's white blood cells

38. _____ rod-shaped bacteria

39. _____ another name for lice

WORD REVIEW

If you do not know the meanings of the words listed below, look them up in the text.

abscesses	hepatitis	pneumonia
acquired immune deficiency syndrome	HIV virus	poisons
	hypodermic needle	pustules
artificially acquired immunity	immune system	rheumatic fever
AIDS	immunity	rickettsia
animal organisms	infection	ringworm
asepsis	influenza	Rocky Mountain spotted fever
bacilli	itch-mite	scabies
bacteria	lice	secretions
blood poisoning	local infection	sepsis
boils	measles	spiral
chicken pox	microbes	spirilla
cilia	microorganisms	spore
cocci	mitosis	staphylococci
common cold	mold	strep throat
corkscrew	mumps	streptococci
diplococci	nail fungus	syphilis
diphtheria	natural immunity	tetanus
disease-causing	naturally acquired immunity	toxins
dormant	nonpathogenic	treponema pallida
flagella	parasites	tuberculosis
fungi	pathogenic	typhoid
fungus	pediculosis	typhus
general infection	plant organisms	vaccine
germs	plant parasite	virus

Sanitation and Disinfection

Date _____

Rating _____

Text Pages 25-36

INTRODUCTION

1. Explain why states have strict rules for sanitation and disinfection procedures.
   _____
   _____

2. a. Define sterilize.
      _____

   b. Define sanitize.
      _____

   c. Between sterilize and sanitize, which one is possible in a salon?
      _____

DISINFECTION

3. Disinfection is almost identical to sterilization but it does not kill _____.
4. Disinfectants control microorganisms on _____ surfaces, but are not safe for use on _____.
5. What items are listed on a Material Safety Data Sheet?
   a. _____
   b. _____
   c. _____
   d. _____
6. List three contaminants that a high-quality disinfectant must destroy.
   a. _____
   b. _____
   c. _____
7. UV sanitizers are useful _____ containers but will not _____ salon implements.
8. Bead "sterilizers" do not _____ implements and are a _____.
9. Formalin contains large amounts of formaldehyde. List five areas of the body it can irritate.
   a. _____

15

b. _____

c. _____

d. _____

e. _____

10. To clean up visible blood, many state cosmetology boards recommend _____.

11. **Matching.** Match the terms on the left with their correct descriptions on the right.

    _____ 1. disinfection container
    _____ 2. quats
    _____ 3. phenolics
    _____ 4. alcohol
    _____ 5. bleach

    A. is extremely flammable and evaporates quickly
    B. best for use when it appears cloudy
    C. the most cost effective of professional disinfectants
    D. best for disinfecting orangewood sticks
    E. can discolor some materials and has almost no cleaning power
    F. a glass, metal, or plastic container used to disinfect implements
    G. has a high alkaline pH level

12. Why should a nail tech have at least two complete sets of implements? _____

13. a. Wash and rinse implements, then immerse them in hospital-level disinfectant for _____.

    b. You and your client should use a _____ on your hands.

PRE-SERVICE SANITATION PROCEDURE

14. A manicuring table should be wiped with a/an _____ solution.

15. How often is the towel that is wrapped on a manicuring cushion to be changed? _____

16. List four manicuring items that are to be discarded after use on one client.

    a. _____

    b. _____

    c. _____

    d. _____

17. What does it mean if the solution in your disinfection container is cloudy? _____

DISINFECTION SAFETY

18. Name two protective items that should be worn when mixing or using disinfectants.

   a. _____
   b. _____

19. List five safety factors in working with disinfectants.

   a. _____
   b. _____
   c. _____
   d. _____
   e. _____

20. List four important factors of Universal Sanitation.

   a. _____
   b. _____
   c. _____
   d. _____

MATCHING REVIEW

Insert the correct word listed in front of each definition below.

alcohol and bleach	formalin	sanitize
antiseptic	moist heat	sanitizers
disinfectant	phenolic	sterilize
disinfection container	quats	ultraviolet ray

21. _____ the most expensive common salon disinfectant
22. _____ effective for storing disinfected implements
23. _____ to destroy all living organisms on an object or surface
24. _____ contains a strong allergic sensitizer
25. _____ to reduce the number of pathogens on a surface
26. _____ cannot be diluted below 70% and remain effective
27. _____ holds a disinfectant solution so items can be submerged
28. _____ a substance that destroys pathogens on implements
29. _____ the common name for quaternary ammonium compounds
30. _____ reduce the number of pathogens in a cut

23. _____ the most expensive common salon disinfectant
24. _____ effective for storing disinfected implements
25. _____ to make something germ-free by destroying all living organisms
26. _____ contains a strong allergic sensitizer
27. _____ to make clean and prevent germs from growing, but is not germfree
28. _____ cannot be diluted below 70% and remain effective
29. _____ holds a disinfectant solution so items can be submerged
30. _____ a chemical agent strong enough to sanitize instruments
31. _____ the common name for quaternary ammonium compound
32. _____ reduce the number of pathogens in a cut

WORD REVIEW

If you do not know the meanings of the words listed below, look them up in the text.

alcohol	disinfection container	quaternary ammonium compound
alkaline	EPA	quats
allergic sensitizer	FDA	residue
antibacterial	formaldehyde	safety glasses
antiseptic	formalin	sanitize
asthma	fungicide	sterilize
bactericide	hepatitis B	tongs
bleach	hospital-level disinfectant	tuberculocidal disinfectant
bronchitis	immersed	ultraviolet ray sanitizer
contaminant	inhalation	Universal Sanitation
corrosion	Material Safety Data Sheet	viricide
decontamination	pH	
disinfectant	phenolics	

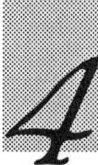

Date _____

Rating _____

Text Pages 37-48

Safety in the Salon

INTRODUCTION

1. None of the products you use as a nail technician _____ to harm your health, but all of them _____ .

COMMON CHEMICALS USED BY NAIL TECHNICIANS

2. List six chemical products commonly found on manicuring tables.
    a. _____
    b. _____
    c. _____
    d. _____
    e. _____
    f. _____

3. Exposure to these chemicals won't harm you, but a danger you need to avoid is _____ .

4. List eleven early warning signs of overexposure to nail chemicals.
    a. _____
    b. _____
    c. _____
    d. _____
    e. _____
    f. _____
    g. _____
    h. _____
    i. _____
    j. _____
    k. _____

LEARN ABOUT THE CHEMICALS IN YOUR PRODUCTS

5. Whose responsibility is it to learn about the chemicals in products and how to handle them safely? _____

6. a. What do the letters MSDS stand for?
   _____

   b. To whom are product manufacturers required to make this sheet available?
   _____

7. List the ten items required on a MSDS.
   a. _____
   b. _____
   c. _____
   d. _____
   e. _____
   f. _____
   g. _____
   h. _____
   i. _____
   j. _____

8. List three ways products can enter your body.
   a. _____
   b. _____
   c. _____

9. The invisible sphere about the size of a beach ball that sits directly in front of your mouth is called your _____ .

10. List four easy and inexpensive ways to eliminate vapors from the salon.
    a. _____
    b. _____
    c. _____
    d. _____

11. The best form of salon vapor and dust control is _____ .

12. To protect your lungs, always wear a _____ when filing or drilling.

HOW TO PROTECT YOURSELF AND YOUR CLIENTS

13. **Figures.** Identify the safety precautions shown in the following figures.

    a. _____

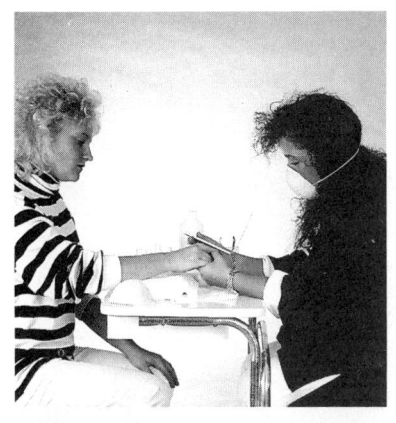

b. _____

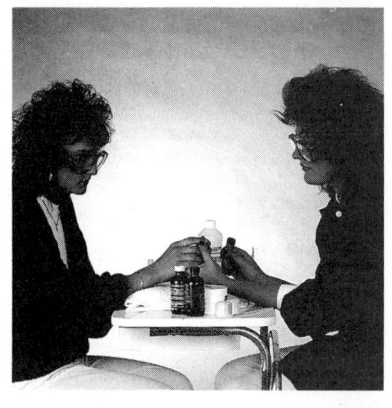

c. _____

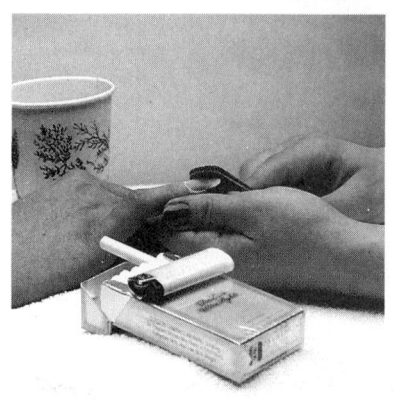

d. _____

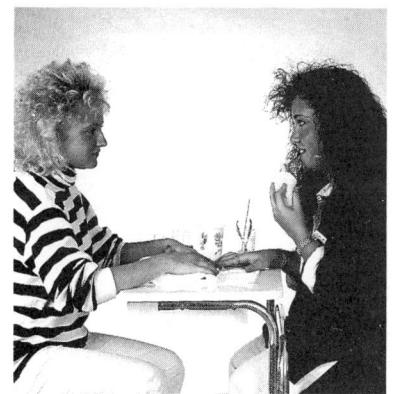

e. _____

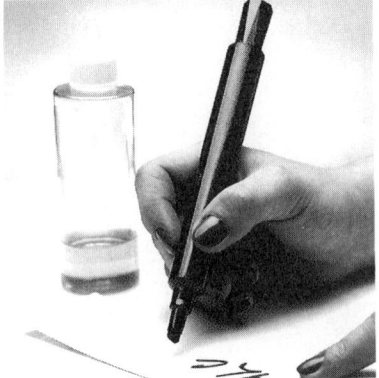

f. _____

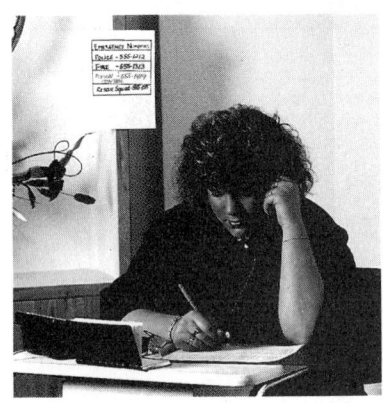

g. _____

14. Explain why you should not store your lunch in the same refrigerator where chemical products are stored.
    _____

15. If you forget to wash your hands before eating, you will probably end up _____ the _____ on your hands.

16. Explain the effect of excessive heat on chemical products.
    _____

17. a. How often should a nail technician's trash be emptied?
    _____ _____

    b. Where should this trash be placed?
    _____

18. What happens to each of the following if you forget to replace its cap?
    a. nail polish: _____
    b. solvents: _____
    c. glue: _____

CUMULATIVE TRAUMA DISORDERS

19. The most common cumulative trauma disorder is _____.

20. Six symptoms of CTDs are:
    a. _____
    b. _____

22

c. _____
d. _____
e. _____
f. _____

MATCHING REVIEW

Insert the correct word listed in front of each definition below.

absorption   glue   overexposure
beauty distributor   local exhaust   solvent
breathing zone   metal container   ventilation
cumulative trauma disorder   MSDS
flammable   nail polish

21. _____ the invisible sphere about the size of a beach ball directly in front of your mouth

22. _____ where you can get MSDS

23. _____ the best form of salon dust and vapor control

24. _____ trash should be placed into this often

25. _____ uncapped, it evaporates

26. _____ Material Safety Data Sheet

27. _____ a system that removes vapors from the salon building

28. _____ early warning signs include watery eyes, light-headedness, and runny nose

29. _____ also known as repetitive motion disorder

30. _____ if left uncapped, it hardens

WORD REVIEW

If you do not know the meanings of the words listed below, look them up in the text.

absorb   expel   MSDS
acrylic liquid   exposure   nail polish
acrylic powder   flammable   overexposure
adhesive dryer   first aid   phenolic disinfectant
breathing zone   gel nail supplies   physical hazards
cancer   glue   poison control center
carcinogen   harmful   polish remover
carpal tunnel syndrome hazards   primer
chemical hazards   HEPA   protection
contaminated   ibuprofen   pump
corrosive   ingestion   repetitive
CTD - Cumulative trauma inhalation   safety glasses
   disorder   insomnia   skin contact
dispose   label   solvents
dust mask   local exhaust   vapors
emergency   manufacturers   ventilation
emergency numbers   Material Safety Data Sheets

23

Part 2

THE SCIENCE OF NAIL TECHNOLOGY

- ◆ *CHAPTER 5* - Nail Product Chemistry Simplified
- ◆ *CHAPTER 6* - Anatomy and Physiology
- ◆ *CHAPTER 7* - The Nail and Its Disorders
- ◆ *CHAPTER 8* - The Skin and Its Disorders
- ◆ *CHAPTER 9* - Client Consultation

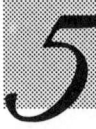

Date _____

Rating _____

Text Pages 50-63

Nail Product Chemistry Simplified

UNDERSTANDING CHEMICALS

1. Almost everything a nail technician does depends on _____.

2. **Matching.** Match the terms on the left with their correct descriptions on the right.

   _____ 1. molecule   A. a molecule that cannot be broken down at all
   _____ 2. matter   B. a change in form or appearance
   _____ 3. chemical change C. something that dissolves another substance
   _____ 4. physical change D. the force that makes two surfaces stick together
   _____ 5. energy   E. something that takes up space and occupies an area
   _____ 6. element   F. a change in chemical substance
                              G. a chemical in its simplest form
                              H. light and microwaves are examples of this

3. A chemical change in a molecule that requires energy to occur is called a _____.

4. A chemical that speeds up a chemical reaction is called a _____.

5. A solvent is something that dissolves another substance, called a _____.

6. The "universal solvent" is _____.

7. A chemical that causes two surfaces to stick together is _____.

8. Primers improve adhesion but can be _____ to soft tissue.

9. Moisture can be temporarily removed from the nail with a _____.

10. List five problems related to overfiling.

    a. _____
    b. _____
    c. _____
    d. _____
    e. _____

FINGERNAIL COATINGS

11. List four common nail coatings.

    a. _____
    b. _____
    c. _____
    d. _____

12. **Matching.** Match the terms on the left with their correct descriptions on the right.

    _____ 1. initiator   A. gigantic chains of molecules
    _____ 2. monomer   B. speeds up a chemical reaction
    _____ 3. cross-linker   C. light-cured enhancements need this
    _____ 4. polymer   D. a monomer that joins different polymer chains
    _____ 5. ultraviolet light E. incandescent light
                                 F. this triggers polymerization
                                 G. examples are nylon, wood, nail plates, hair

AVOIDING SKIN PROBLEMS

13. Skin inflammation is called _____ .

14. List two types of contact dermatitis.

    a. _____
    b. _____

15. List four likely places for allergies to occur.

    a. _____
    b. _____
    c. _____
    d. _____

16. Overexposure refers to _____.

17. List four things that cause gels to harden incorrectly, therefore, causing skin problems.

    a. _____
    b. _____
    c. _____
    d. _____

18. Chemicals that enlarge the vessels around an injury are called _____.

19. A common salon irritant is _____.

20. Symptoms of contact dermatitis are isolated to _____.

MATCHING REVIEW

Insert the correct word listed in front of each definition below.

adhesive   initiator   polymer
catalyst   matter   solute
contact dermatitis molecule   solvent
cross-linker   monomer
histamine   overexposure

21. _____ a chemical in its simplest form
22. _____ something that dissolves another substance
23. _____ skin inflammation caused by touching certain substances to the skin
24. _____ a gigantic chain of molecules
25. _____ takes up space or occupies an area
26. _____ chemical that enlarges the vessels around an injury
27. _____ prolonged, repeated, long-term exposure
28. _____ something that speeds a chemical reaction
29. _____ a monomer that joins polymer chains
30. _____ a chemical that causes two surfaces to stick together

WORD REVIEW

If you do not know the meanings of the words listed below, look them up in the text.

abrasive   dehydrator   molecule
acetone   dermatitis   monomer
adhesion   element   overexposure
adhesive   energy   pigment
alchemist   epidermis   polymer
allergic   evaporate   polymerization
catalyst   flammable   primer
chemical   glue   saturate
chemical change   histamine   sensitization
chemical reaction   incandescent   simple polymer chain
contaminate   incompatible   solute
coatings   initiator   solvent
contact dermatitis irritant   substance
corrosive   matter   ultraviolet (UV) light
cross-linker   medieval   universal solvent
cyanoacrylate   microwave   volatile

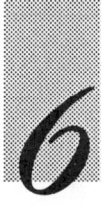

Date _____

Rating _____

Text Pages 64-85

Anatomy and Physiology

INTRODUCTION

1. Explain why a nail technician must study anatomy and physiology.
   _____

2. List four parts of the human body.
   a. _____
   b. _____
   c. _____
   d. _____

CELLS

3. Define cells.
   _____

4. **Matching.** Match the terms on the left with their correct descriptions on the right.

   _____ 1. cytoplasm   A. a small round body in the cytoplasm
   _____ 2. cell membrane   B. groups of cells of the same kind
   _____ 3. protoplasm   C. a colorless, jellylike substance
   _____ 4. centrosome   D. found in the center of the cell
   _____ 5. nucleus   E. encloses the cytoplasm
                              F. found outside of a cell
                              G. found outside the nucleus
                              H. a colorful, jellylike substance

CELL GROWTH

5. Under what three conditions will a cell continue to grow?
   a. _____
   b. _____
   c. _____

6. Cells reproduce themselves through a process of cell division called _____ .

7. **Identification.** Using the letters **M, A,** and **C** (defined below), match the correct characteristics below.

Key:

M = metabolism
A = anabolism
C = catabolism

Characteristics:

_____ a. stores water, food, and oxygen
_____ b. complex process where cells are nourished and supplied with energy
_____ c. breaks down larger molecules into smaller ones
_____ d. builds up larger molecules from smaller ones
_____ e. has two phases
_____ f. releases energy for muscle contraction, secretion, or heat production

8. Define homeostasis.
_____

9. a. Explain why people gain weight.
_____

   b. Explain how people can get rid of fat.
_____

TISSUES

10. Define tissue.
_____

11. **Matching.** Match the terms on the left with their correct descriptions on the right.

    _____ 1. connective   A. basic unit of all living things
    _____ 2. muscular   B. carries message to and from the brain
    _____ 3. nerve   C. anabolism and catabolism
    _____ 4. epithelial   D. supports, protects, and binds together other body tissues
    _____ 5. liquid
                                    E. a protective covering on body surfaces
                                    F. maintains homeostasis
                                    G. contracts and moves various parts of the body
                                    H. carries food, waste products, hormones

ORGANS

12. Define organs.
_____

13. **Matching.** Match the terms on the left with their correct descriptions on the right.

   _____ 1. brain
   _____ 2. heart
   _____ 3. lungs
   _____ 4. kidneys
   _____ 5. stomach

   A. supplies oxygen to the blood
   B. a storage place for unused fat cells
   C. excretes water and other wastes
   D. part of the reproductive system
   E. controls the body
   F. digests food
   G. circulates the blood
   H. encloses the protoplasm
   I. removes toxic products of digestion

SYSTEMS

14. a. Define systems.

   _____

   b. How many systems are in the body?

   _____

15. **Matching.** Match the systems on the left with their correct descriptions on the right.

   _____ 1. integumentary
   _____ 2. skeletal
   _____ 3. muscular
   _____ 4. nervous
   _____ 5. circulatory
   _____ 6. endocrine
   _____ 7. excretory
   _____ 8. respiratory
   _____ 9. digestive
   _____ 10. reproductive

   A. supplies oxygen to the body
   B. produces all body movements
   C. made up of duct glands
   D. supplies blood through the body
   E. the skin's dermis and epidermis
   F. made up of nucleus, centrosome, and cell membrane
   G. enables human beings to reproduce
   H. changes food into usable substances
   I. the bones of the body
   J. anabolism and catabolism are part of this
   K. controls and coordinates the functions of all other body systems
   L. eliminates waste from the body
   M. made up of ductless glands

OVERVIEW OF ANATOMY AND PHYSIOLOGY

16. Define anatomy.

   _____

17. Define physiology.

   _____

   _____

THE SKELETAL SYSTEM

18. How many bones are on a skeleton?
    _____

19. Bone is the _____ tissue of the body.

20. Define osteology.
    _____

21. The technical term for bone is _____.

22. List five functions of bones.

    a. _____
    b. _____
    c. _____
    d. _____
    e. _____

23. **Matching.** Match the terms on the left with their correct descriptions on the right.

    _____ 1. periosteum
    _____ 2. cartilage
    _____ 3. ligaments
    _____ 4. synovial fluid
    _____ 5. pivot joint
    _____ 6. hinge joint
    _____ 7. ball and socket joint
    _____ 8. gliding joints

    A. two or more bones connect like a door
    B. lubricates at the joints
    C. another name for collar bone
    D. cushions bone at the joints
    E. rounded bone fits into the hollow of another bone
    F. a fibrous membrane that covers and protects the bone
    G. one bone turns on another bone
    H. also called osteology
    I. two bones glide over each other
    J. bands or sheets of fibrous tissue that support bones at the joints
    K. technical term for bone

24. Another name for the collar bone is _____ .

25. The fingers, or _____ have three _____ in each finger and two in the thumb.

26. Figure 6.3: Label the bones of the arm and hand.

27. Figure 6.5 and 6.6: Label the bones of the leg and foot.

28. Similar to the finger bones, the bones of the toes are called _____ . There are two of these in the big toe and _____ in the other toes.

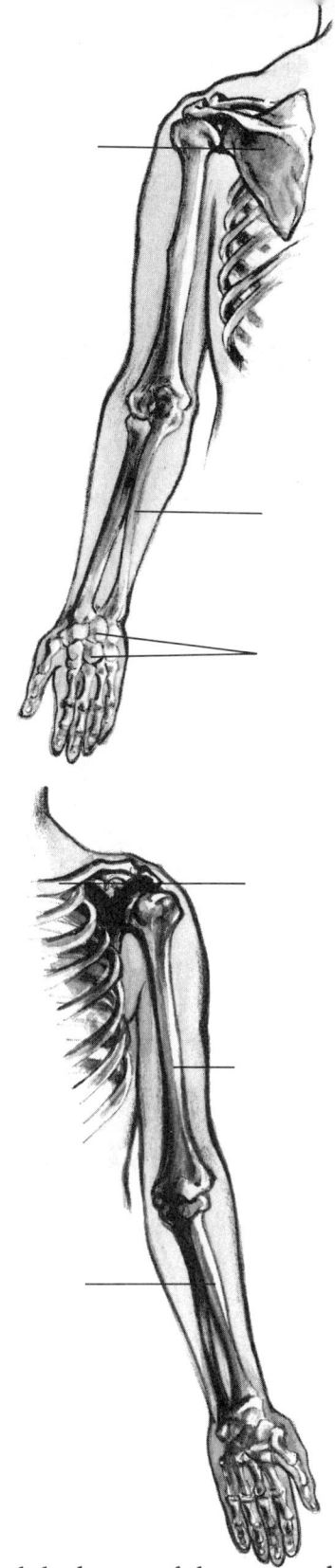

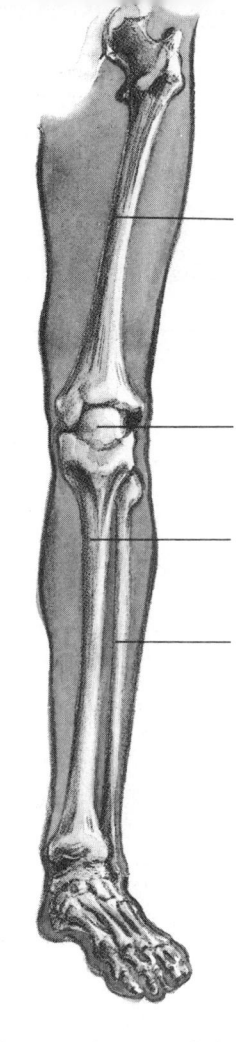

Label the bones of the leg.

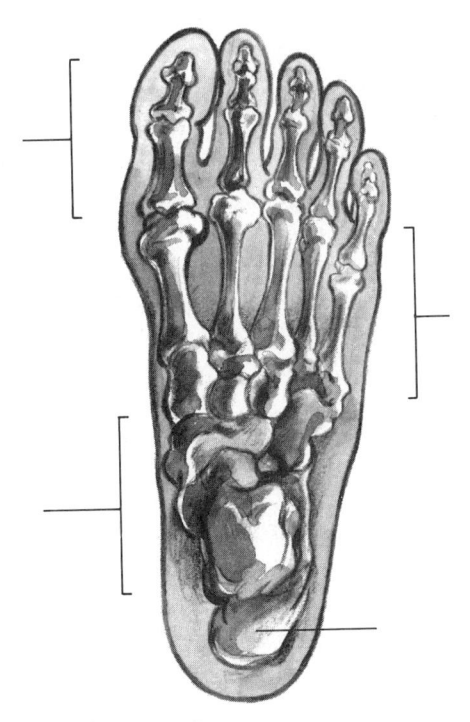

Label the bones of the arm and hand.

Label the bones of the foot.

33

THE MUSCULAR SYSTEM

29. Define myology.
_____

30. a. How many muscles are in the body?
_____

   b. What percent of body weight does the muscular system comprise?
_____

31. Define muscles.
_____

32. **Matching.** Match the terms on the left with their correct descriptions on the right.

   _____ 1. striated   A. muscle part that moves
   _____ 2. non-striated   B. heart muscle
   _____ 3. cardiac   C. infrared and ultraviolet are examples
   _____ 4. origin   D. voluntary muscles
   _____ 5. insertion   E. also called phalanges
   _____ 6. belly   F. can be performed by hand or electric vibrator
   _____ 7. massage   G. middle part of a muscle
   _____ 8. electric current H. muscles of the hand
   _____ 9. light rays   I. involuntary muscles
   _____ 10. heat rays   J. also called digits
   _____ 11. moist heat   K. lamps and caps produce these
                               L. applied to muscle to produce visible muscle contractions
                               M. muscle part that does not move
                               N. example is steam

33. Explain how pressure is usually directed when massage is performed.
_____

34. **Identification.** Using the letters **A, F, H,** and **L** (defined below), match the following muscles with the correct part of the body.

   Key:
   A = shoulder and upper arm muscles
   F = forearm muscles
   H = hand muscles
   L = lower leg and foot muscles

   Muscles:
   _____ a. flexor
   _____ b. extensor digitorum longus
   _____ c. extensor

34

_____ d. adductors

_____ e. biceps

_____ f. peroneus longus

_____ g. gastrocnemius

_____ h. supinator

_____ i. flexor digitorum brevis

_____ j. abductors

_____ k. peroneus brevis

_____ l. deltoid

_____ m. abductor hallucis

_____ n. tibialis anterior

_____ o. pronator

_____ p. opponent

_____ q. triceps

_____ r. soleus

THE NERVOUS SYSTEM

35. Define neurology.

   _____

36. Explain the purpose of the nervous system.

   _____

   _____

37. **Identification.** Using the letters **C, P,** and **A** (defined below), match the characteristics below with the three divisions of the nervous system.

   Key:

   C = central nervous system

   P = peripheral nervous system

   A = automatic nervous system

   Characteristics:

   _____ a. made up of sensory and motor nerve fibers

   _____ b. functions without conscious effort

   _____ c. consists of the brain and spinal cord

   _____ d. has sympathetic and parasympathetic systems

   _____ e. controls the five senses

   _____ f. carries messages to and from the central nervous system

   _____ g. also called the cerebro-spinal nervous system

   _____ h. regulates activities of the glands and heart

   _____ i. controls all mental activities

35

THE BRAIN AND SPINAL CORD

38. The brain is the body's largest mass of _____ tissue and is contained in the _____ . It weighs _____ ounces.

39. a. Where does the spinal cord originate?
    _____

    b. How many pairs of nerves extend from the spinal cord?
    _____

NERVE CELLS AND NERVES

40. Define nerves.
    _____
    _____

41. **Matching.** Match the terms on the left with their correct descriptions on the right.

    _____ 1. neuron
    _____ 2. dendrites
    _____ 3. axon
    _____ 4. sensory nerves
    _____ 5. motor nerves
    _____ 6. mixed nerves
    _____ 7. receptors
    _____ 8. reflex

    A. sends messages to other neurons, glands or muscles
    B. also called ulnar
    C. have ability to send and receive messages
    D. automatic response to a stimulus
    E. also called afferent nerves
    F. has sympathetic and parasympathetic systems
    G. primary structural unit of the nervous system
    H. sensory nerve endings
    I. the body's largest mass of nerve tissue
    J. a cell body that receives messages from other neurons
    K. also called efferent nerves

NERVES OF THE ARM AND HAND

42. Label nerves of the arm and hand.

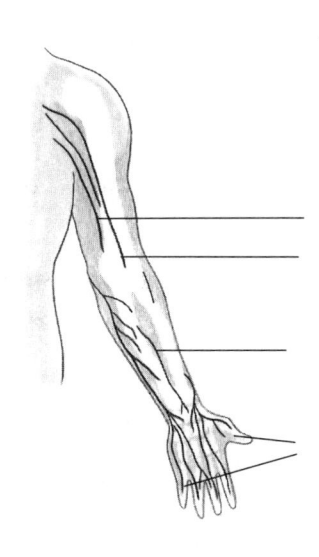

NERVES OF THE LOWER LEG AND FOOT

43. List seven nerves of the lower leg and foot.

   a. _____
   b. _____
   c. _____
   d. _____
   e. _____
   f. _____
   g. _____

THE CIRCULATORY SYSTEM

44. a. What is another name for the circulatory system?
   _____

   b. List two systems within the vascular system.

   1. _____
   2. _____

THE HEART

45. What is the heart?
   _____

46. The heart is enclosed in a membrane called the _____.

47. How many times does the heart beat at the normal resting rate?
   _____

48. List the four chambers of the heart.

   a. _____
   b. _____
   c. _____
   d. _____

49. Tubes that carry blood from the heart are _____ and those that carry blood to the heart are _____.

50. What allows blood to flow in only one direction?
   _____

THE BLOOD

51. Define blood.
   _____
   _____

52. Blood's normal temperature is _____.

53. How many pints of blood are in an adult?

54. Explain why blood changes color from bright to dark red.

55. List two types of blood circulation.

    a. _____

    b. _____

56. **Matching.** Match the terms on the left with their correct descriptions on the right.

    _____ 1. pulmonary   A. carry oxygen to the cells
    _____ 2. white corpuscles B. help the blood to clot
    _____ 3. plasma   C. circulation from the heart to the lungs
    _____ 4. red corpuscles   D. equalizes body temperature
    _____ 5. systemic   E. fluid part of the blood
    _____ 6. blood platelets F. main blood supply to the hand
                                G. circulation from the heart through the body and back to the heart
                                H. tubes that carry blood to the heart
                                I. destroy disease-causing germs

57. List six arteries that supply blood for the arms, hands, lower leg, and foot.

    a. _____
    b. _____
    c. _____
    d. _____
    e. _____
    f. _____

THE LYMPH-VASCULAR SYSTEM

58. Define lymph.

59. Explain five functions of lymph.

    a. _____
    b. _____
    c. _____
    d. _____
    e. _____

THE ENDOCRINE SYSTEM

60. Define gland.

_____

61. What substance(s) do the endocrine glands secrete?

_____

THE EXCRETORY SYSTEM

62. Explain how the excretory system purifies the body.

_____

63. List five body organs that are a part of this system. After each, list what waste matter that organ eliminates.

   Organ: **Waste Matter:**

   1. _____   _____
   2. _____   _____
   3. _____   _____
   4. _____   _____
   5. _____   _____

THE RESPIRATORY SYSTEM

64. a. Spongy tissues composed of microscopic cells that take in air are called _____.

   b. A muscular partition that controls breathing is called the _____.

65. a. The gas we inhale is _____.

   b. The gas we exhale is _____.

THE DIGESTIVE SYSTEM

66. Define digestion.

_____

67. a. Where does digestion begin?

   _____

   b. Where does it end?

   _____

   c. List three organs between the mouth and small intestine.

   a. _____
   b. _____
   c. _____

68. The large intestine, also called the _____, stores refuse for elimination through the _____.

69. How long does the complete digestive process take?

_____

39

70. Define digestive enzymes.
   _____
   _____

71. **Identification.** Using the letters, **S, M, N, C, EN, EX, R,** and **D** (defined below), match the correct characteristics below with one of the body's ten systems.

   Key:
   S   = skeletal system
   M   = muscular system
   N   = nervous system
   C   = circulatory system
   EN = endocrine system
   EX = excretory system
   R   = respiratory system
   D   = digestive system

   Characteristics:

   _____ a. ductless glands
   _____ b. makes up 40%-50% of body weight
   _____ c. cleans the body by eliminating waste
   _____ d. supplies oxygen to the body
   _____ e. central, peripheral, and autonomic
   _____ f. converts food so the body can use it
   _____ g. also called the vascular system
   _____ h. lungs take in air
   _____ i. pharynx, esophagus, and stomach
   _____ j. the study of this is osteology
   _____ k. urine from the kidneys
   _____ l. secretes hormones
   _____ m. diaphragm controls breathing
   _____ n. bile from the liver
   _____ o. origin, belly, and insertion
   _____ p. begins in the mouth, ends in the small intestine
   _____ q. digits and phalanges
   _____ r. glands in it secrete substances
   _____ s. the study of this is neurology
   _____ t. two types are blood-vascular and lymph-vascular
   _____ u. veins, arteries, corpuscles, and lymph-vascular
   _____ v. the study of this is myology
   _____ w. neurons, sensory, and reflexes
   _____ x. joints, periosteum, and ligaments

WORD REVIEW

If you do not know the meanings of the words listed below, look them up in the text.

abductors
abductor hallucis
adductors
afferent nerves
anabolism
anatomy
anterior tibial artery
arteries
auricle
autonomic nervous system
axon and axon terminal
ball-and-socket joint
belly
biceps
blood
blood platelets
blood-vascular system
bones
brain
calcaneous
capillaries
carbon dioxide
cardiac
carpus/wrist
cartilage
catabolism
cell(s)
cell membrane
central nervous system
centrosome
cerebro-spinal nervous system
circulatory system
clavicle
common peroneal nerve
connective tissue
cytoplasm
deep peroneal nerve
deltoid
dendrites
diaphragm
digestion
digestive enzymes
digestive system
digital nerve
digits
dorsalis pedis artery
dorsal nerve
ductless glands

efferent nerves
electric current
endocrine system
enzymes
epithelial tissue
erythrocytes
esophagus
excretory system
exhale
extensor
extensor digatorum brevis
extensor digitorum longus
femur
fibula
flexor
flexor digatorum brevis
forearm
gastrocnemius
glands
gliding joints
heart
heat rays
hinge joints
homeostasis
hormones
humerus
inhale
insertion
integumentary system
intestines
joints
kidneys
lacteals
left atrium
left ventricle
leucocytes
ligaments
light rays
liquid tissue
liver
lungs
lymph
lymphatic system
lymph glands
lymph-vascular system
massage
median nerve
metabolism
metacarpals

metatarsals
mitosis
mixed nerves
moist heat
motor nerves
muscular system
muscular tissue
myology
neurology
nerve tissue
nerves
nervous system
neuron
non-striated
nucleus
opponent
organs
origin
os
osteology
oxygen
parasympathetic system
patella
pericardium
peripheral system
periosteum
peroneus brevis
peroneus longus
perspiration
phalanges
pharynx
physiology
pivot joints
plasma
popliteal artery
posterior tibial artery
pronator
protoplasm
pulmonary circulation
radial artery
radial nerve
radius
receptors
red corpuscles
reflex
reproductive system
respiratory system
right atrium
right ventricle

saphenous nerve
scapula
sensory nerves
sinews
skeletal system
soleus
spinal cord
stomach
striated
superficial peroneal nerve
supinator

sural nerve
sympathetic system
synovial fluid
systemic circulation
systems
tarsal
tendons
tibia
tibial nerve
tibialis anterior
tissues

triceps
ulna
ulnar artery
ulnar nerve
urine
vagus
valves
vascular system
veins
white corpuscles

7

Date _____

Rating _____

Text Pages 86-95

The Nail and Its Disorders

INTRODUCTION

1. List three characteristics of healthy nails.

   a. _____

   b. _____

   c. _____

2. What is the technical term for nail?
   _____

3. a. The name of the protein nails are made of is
   _____

   b. List two other things that are made of the same protein.

      1. _____

      2. _____

4. Explain why we have nails.
   _____

5. a. How fast do fingernails grow?
   _____

   b. The season of the year when nails grow faster is _____.

   c. The finger that has the slowest growing nail is the _____. The finger with the fastest growing nail is the _____ finger.

   d. If a person has lost an entire nail (through disease or accident), how long will it take for the nail to replace itself?
   _____

PARTS OF THE NAIL

6. Label the parts of the nail.

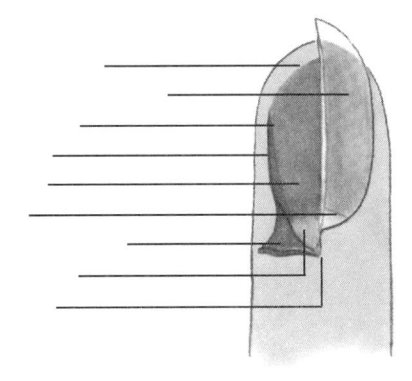

43

7. **Matching.** Match the nail parts of the left with their correct descriptions on the right.

    _____ 1. body/plate
    _____ 2. nail fold (mantle)
    _____ 3. lunula
    _____ 4. wall
    _____ 5. root
    _____ 6. perionychium
    _____ 7. free edge
    _____ 8. grooves
    _____ 9. hyponychium
    _____ 10. matrix
    _____ 11. eponychium
    _____ 12. nail bed
    _____ 13. cuticle

    A. deep fold of skin at nail base
    B. thin line of skin from nail wall to plate
    C. skin beneath nail plate/body
    D. skin under the free edge
    E. skin on sides above grooves
    F. main nail part constructed in layers
    G. bottom skin of each toe
    H. contains nerves and blood; if injured, irregular nail forms
    I. nail grows along these tracks
    J. overlapping skin around nail
    K. bottom skin of each finger
    L. extends beyond the fingertip
    M. where nail growth begins
    N. nails are made of this protein
    O. half-moon shape at nail base
    P. skin surrounding entire nail

NAIL DISORDERS

8. Define nail disorder.
   _____

9. To make a responsible decision about whether you should perform a service on a client, a nail technician must learn to recognize the _____ of nail disorders.

10. List and describe four symptoms of the nail or skin on which a nail technician should **not** work.

    Symptom:　　　　　　　　　　　　**Description:**
    a. _____　　_____
    b. _____　　_____
    c. _____　　_____
    d. _____　　_____
    　　　　　　　　　　　　　　　　_____

44

NAIL DISORDERS THAT CAN BE SERVICED BY A NAIL TECHNICIAN

11. **Matching.** Match the terms on the left with their correct descriptions on the right.

    _____ 1. furrows or corrugations
    _____ 2. onychophagy
    _____ 3. discolored nails
    _____ 4. onychatrophia or atrophy
    _____ 5. pterygium
    _____ 6. onychorrhexis
    _____ 7. onychocryptosis or ingrown nails
    _____ 8. agnails or hangnails
    _____ 9. leukonychia
    _____ 10. onychauxis or hypertrophy
    _____ 11. eggshell nails

    A. split or brittle nails
    B. cuticle is dry, so it splits
    C. fungus infection with blisters
    D. fragile thin, white, and curved nails
    E. common forward cuticle growth
    F. bitten, deformed nails
    G. long depressions that run lengthwise or across the nail
    H. plate loosens, does not fall or come off
    I. nail appears blue in color
    J. the overgrowth of nails
    K. nail grows into the tissue on the sides of the nail
    L. wasting away of the nail
    M. white spots on the nail
    N. bacterial infection of the tissue around the nail

12. How can a nail technician correct agnails (hangnails)?
    _____

13. List two things that can be applied to hide discolored nails.
    a. _____
    b. _____

14. Because eggshell nails are fragile and break easily, filing should be done with the _____ side of an emery board. Using a metal pusher at the base of the nail should not be done with much _____.

15. What type of pusher should be used when manicuring a client who has furrows on their nails?
    _____

16. List three causes of leukonychia.
    a. _____
    b. _____
    c. _____

45

17. Three things that happen to a nail with onychatrophia, or atrophy, are that it loses its
    _____ , it _____ , and falls _____ .

18. File an onychauxis, or hypertropy, nail _____ and buff it with
    _____.

19. a. List two causes of onychocryptosis.
    1. _____
    2. _____

    b. If the tissue around the onychocryptosis nail is not infected, you can trim the nail corner in a curved shape to relieve the _____ on the nail groove.

    c. If the onychocryptosis nail has grown deeply into the groove, refer the client to a _____ .

20. Describe how the condition onychophagy can be improved.
    _____

21. a. List four causes of onychorrhexis.
    1. _____
    2. _____
    3. _____
    4. _____

    b. Discuss two ways onychorrhexis can be corrected.
    1. _____
    2. _____

22. Explain how pterygium can be treated.
    _____
    _____

23. a. List seven causes of corrugations.
    1. _____
    2. _____
    3. _____
    4. _____
    5. _____
    6. _____
    7. _____

    b. Discuss how the appearance of corrugations can be corrected if the ridges are not deep and the nail is not broken.
    _____
    _____

NAIL DISORDERS THAT CANNOT BE SERVICED BY A NAIL TECHNICIAN

24. **Matching.** Match the terms on the left with their correct descriptions on the right.

   _____ 1. onychomycosis tinea unguium
   _____ 2. onycholysis
   _____ 3. pyogenic granuloma
   _____ 4. onychia
   _____ 5. paronychia
   _____ 6. mold
   _____ 7. onychoptosis
   _____ 8. onychogryposis

   A. severe inflammation of nail; red tissue grows from nail bed to nail plate
   B. turns from yellow-green into black
   C. nail becomes thicker and curves, sometimes over the nail tip
   D. plate loosens from nail bed
   E. inflammation in the nail
   F. white spots on the nail plate
   G. periodically, part or all of the nail sheds and falls off
   H. ingrown nails
   I. nail biting
   J. bacterial inflammation of tissue around the nail
   K. infectious disease caused by a fungus; three forms

25. **Identification.** Using the letters **Y** and **N** (defined below) answer the following question: Can a nail technician perform a service on the following nail disorders?

   Key:
   Y = yes, a service can be performed on this disorder
   N = no, a service cannot be performed on this disorder

   Disorders:

   _____ a. leukonychia
   _____ b. onychatrophia
   _____ c. onychia
   _____ d. eggshell nails
   _____ e. onychomycosis tinea unguium
   _____ f. onychoptosis
   _____ g. onychophagy
   _____ h. paronychia
   _____ i. furrows
   _____ j. onychogryposis
   _____ k. onychauxis

   _____ l. onychophyma
   _____ m. onychocryptosis
   _____ n. onycholysis
   _____ o. discolored nails
   _____ p. pterygium
   _____ q. mold
   _____ r. nevus
   _____ s. agnails
   _____ t. onychorrhexis
   _____ u. pyogenic granuloma

47

26. Below each figure, label the disorder shown.

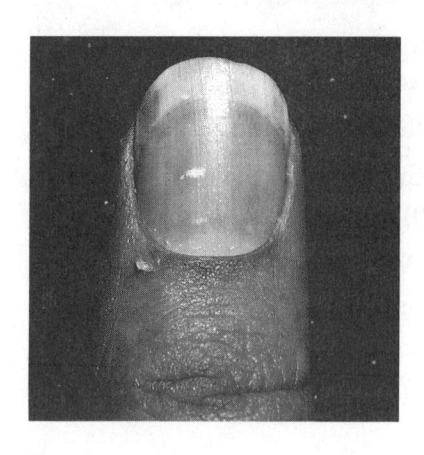

a. _____

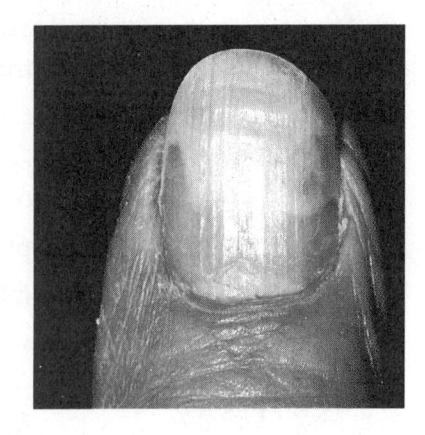

b. _____

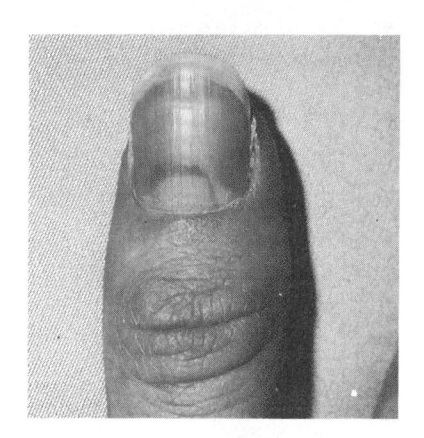

c. _____

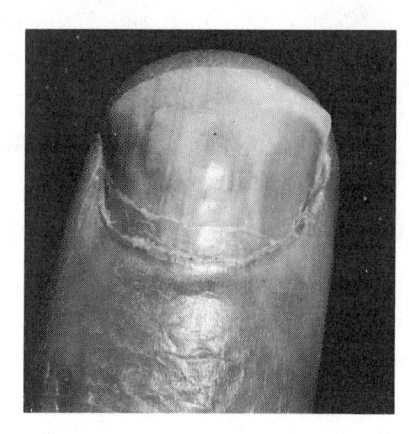

d. _____

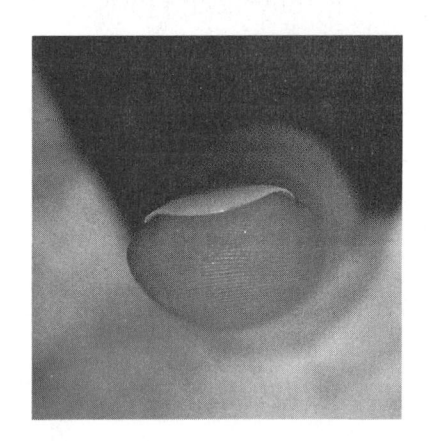

e. _____

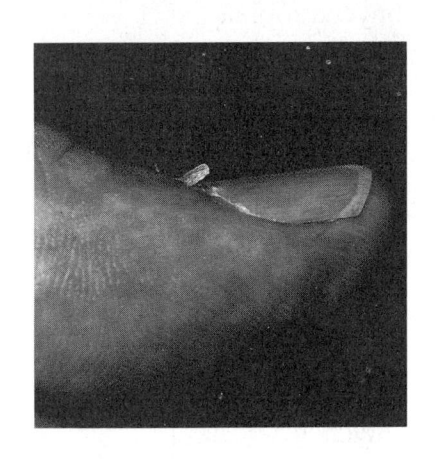

f. _____

48

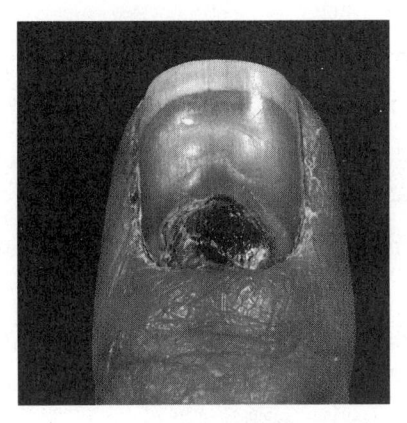

g. _____

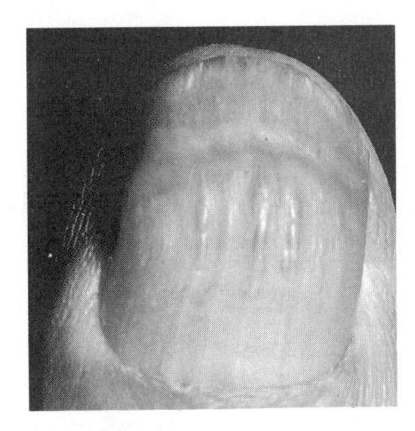

h. _____

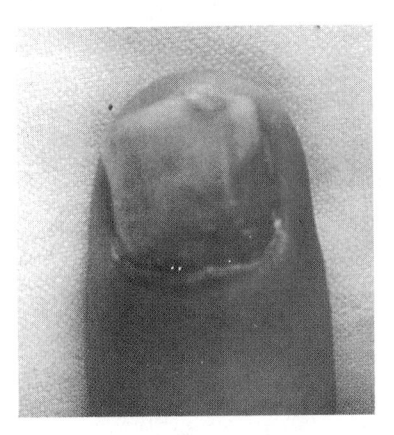

i. _____

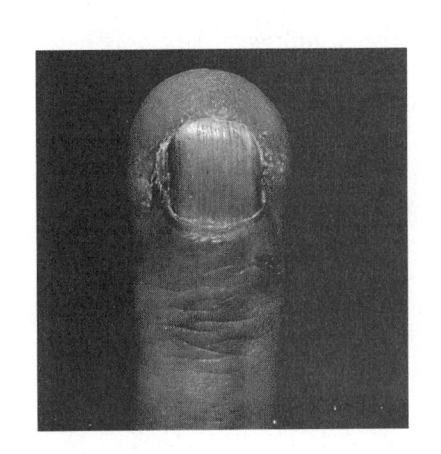

j. _____

MATCHING REVIEW

Insert the correct word listed in front of each definition below.

cuticle			matrix			onychophagy
hangnails		nail body/plate		onycholysis
hyponychium		nail root		onyx
keratin			onychia			paronychia
leukonychia		onychocryptosis		pterygium
lunula			onychogryposis

27. _____ technical term for nail
28. _____ cuticle splits because of dryness
29. _____ overlapping skin around the nail
30. _____ where nail growth begins
31. _____ white spots on the nail
32. _____ main nail part constructed in layers

49

33. _____ nails are made out of this protein
34. _____ nail plate loosens from the nail bed
35. _____ nail biting
36. _____ half-moon shape at the base of the nail
37. _____ part of skin under the free edge
38. _____ ingrown nails
39. _____ contains nerves and blood; if it is injured, an irregular nail will form
40. _____ an inflammation somewhere in the nail

WORD REVIEW

If you do not know the meanings of the words listed below, look them up in the text.

broken skin	leukonychia	onychocryptosis
bruised nails	lunula	onychogryposis
corrugations	mantle	onychomycosis
cuticle	matrix	onycholysis
dermatologist	mold	onychophagy
discolored nails	nail bed	onychophyma
eggshell nails	nail body/plate	onychoptosis
eponychium	nail disorder	onychorrhexis
free edge	nail fold	onyx
furrows	nail grooves	paronychia
hangnails (agnails)	nail root	perionychium
hyponychium	nail wall(s)	pterygium
infection	nevus	pyogenic granuloma
inflammation	onychatrophia (atrophy)	raised/swollen skin
ingrown nails	onychauxis (hypertrophy)	
keratin	onychia	

8

Date _____

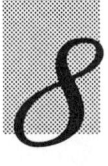

Rating _____

Text Pages 96-106

The Skin and Its Disorders

INTRODUCTION

1. Why must a nail technician have a basic understanding of the skin?
   _____

2. Explain two reasons why knowledge of the skin will help you
   a. _____
   b. _____

HEALTHY SKIN

3. Define dermatology.
   _____

4. List four characteristics of healthy skin.
   a. _____   c. _____
   b. _____   d. _____

5. a. Where is our skin the thickest?   b. Where is our skin the thinnest?
   _____   _____

FUNCTIONS OF THE SKIN

6. **Matching.** Match the terms on the left with their correct descriptions on the right.

   _____ 1. protection
   _____ 2. secretion
   _____ 3. absorption
   _____ 4. prevention of fluid loss
   _____ 5. respiration
   _____ 6. heat regulation
   _____ 7. excretion
   _____ 8. response to external stimuli

   A. skin seals blood and other fluids inside the body
   B. sudoriferous gland records hot, cold, pain, and pleasure
   C. maintain 98.6° F
   D. skin's shield from injury and bacteria invasion
   E. oxygen taken in and carbon dioxide is discharged
   F. pores take in small amounts of chemicals, drugs, and cosmetics
   G. sebum eliminates wastes
   H. skin's sensitivity to heat, cold, touch, pressure, and pain
   I. carbon dioxide taken in and oxygen is discharged
   J. perspiration removes salt and other wastes
   K. sebum slows moisture evaporation

7. Label the microscopic section of the skin.

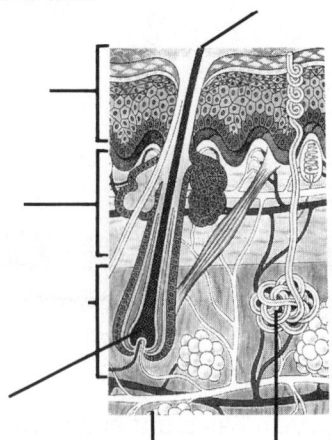

8. **Identification.** Using the letters **E** and **D** (defined below), match the characteristics below with one of the skin layers.

   Key:
   E = epidermis
   D = dermis

   Characteristics:

   _____ 1. contains three separate layers
   _____ 2. blood vessels, nerves, sweat, and oil glands are found in this layer
   _____ 3. also called cuticle or scarf skin
   _____ 4. made up of four layers called stratums
   _____ 5. deep layer of the skin
   _____ 6. papillary, reticular, and subcutaneous
   _____ 7. melanin is found here
   _____ 8. contains nerve endings, but no blood vessels
   _____ 9. adipose tissue is found here
   _____ 10. outer layer of the skin
   _____ 11. also called true skin, corium, or cutis
   _____ 12. keratin is found here

9. List four layers of the epidermis.

   a. _____
   b. _____
   c. _____
   d. _____

10. a. The name of the skin coloring pigment is _____.
    b. The special cells that make the skin coloring pigment are found in the stratum _____.

c. The skin coloring pigment protects the body from the destructive effects of _____ rays.

11. a. List the layers of the dermis.

    1. _____
    2. _____
    3. _____

    b. Which layer of the dermis is directly below the epidermis?
    _____

12. a. Which layer of the dermis is made of fatty tissue?
    _____

    b. Another name for the fatty tissue is _____ .

    c. Explain three purposes or functions of this fatty tissue.

    1. _____
    2. _____
    3. _____

NOURISHMENT OF THE SKIN

13. What is lymph?
    _____

14. List three parts of a network through which blood and lymph circulate through the skin.

    a. _____
    b. _____
    c. _____

15. For what three things do the blood and lymph supply growth and repair nourishment?

    a. _____
    b. _____
    c. _____

NERVES OF THE SKIN

16. Explain the action(s) of nerves.
    _____
    _____

17. a. List three types of nerves.

    1. _____
    2. _____
    3. _____

    b. Which type of nerve causes goose bumps?
    _____

    c. The nerves of the sweat and oil glands are called _____ nerves.

d. Which type of nerve reacts to touch?
_____

GLANDS OF THE SKIN

18. a. The skin contains two types of _____ glands.

    b. Explain what duct glands do to materials from the blood.
    _____

    c. List two actions that may happen to these different materials from the blood.
       1. _____
       2. _____

19. **Identification.** Using the letters **SU** and **SE** (defined below), match the correct characteristics below with one type of gland.

    Key:
    SU = sudoriferous gland
    SE = sebaceous gland

    Characteristics:

    _____ a. eliminates 1-2 pints of liquids daily
    _____ b. not found on the palms or soles
    _____ c. regulates body temperature
    _____ d. also called oil glands
    _____ e. lubricates skin and softens hair
    _____ f. palms, soles, forehead, and armpits have the greatest amount of them
    _____ g. a blackhead may form
    _____ h. also called sweat glands
    _____ i. has a coiled base called a fundus
    _____ j. opens into the hair follicle
    _____ k. secretes sebum
    _____ l. eliminates waste products

ELASTICITY OF THE SKIN

20. Explain the action of the elastic tissue in the papillary layer.
    _____
    _____

21. Why does skin sag or wrinkle?
    _____

SKIN DISORDERS

22. Explain why nail technicians need to learn about skin disorders.
    _____
    _____

23. The only person qualified to diagnose a disorder/disease is a _____.

24. List four skin symptoms that indicate that disease is present.

   a. _____
   b. _____
   c. _____
   d. _____

25. Define lesion.
   _____
   _____

26. Label the skin lesions shown in the diagram.

27. Describe the following lesions.

   a. cyst: _____
   _____

   b. macule: _____
   _____

   c. papule: _____
   _____

   d. pustule: _____
   _____

   e. tubercle: _____
   _____

   f. tumor: _____
   _____

28. **Matching.** Match the terms on the left with their correct descriptions on the right.

        _____ 1. excoriation
        _____ 2. scales
        _____ 3. vesicle
        _____ 4. crust
        _____ 5. stain
        _____ 6. ulcer
        _____ 7. fissure
        _____ 8. bulla
        _____ 9. wheals (hives)
        _____ 10. scar

    A. bug bites or allergic reactions cause these
    B. example is severe dandruff
    C. an open lesion on the skin
    D. a scab on a sore, for example
    E. a light colored raised mark formed after an injury has healed
    F. fluid lump above and below the skin's surface
    G. poison ivy produces these small blisters
    H. abnormal cell mass that varies in size, shape, and color
    I. large blister with watery fluid
    J. scratching causes this sore or abrasion
    K. discoloration remains after moles, freckles, or liver spots have disappeared
    L. chapped hands or lips are examples
    M. small pimple that does not contain fluid

INFLAMMATION OF THE SKIN

29. Another name for skin inflammation is _____.

30. a. List two skin inflammations.

    1. _____
    2. _____

    b. How long lasting are the two skin inflammations in question 30a?
    _____

    c. Which skin inflammation has dry patches and silvery scales?
    _____

    d. Which skin inflammation itches, burns, and has oozing blisters?
    _____

    e. Which skin inflammation is rarely found on the face?
    _____

INFECTIONS, PIGMENTATION, HYPERTROPIES OF THE SKIN

31. Describe two factors that determine the skin's color.

    a. _____

    b. _____

32. Define hypertropies.

    _____

33. A nail technician cannot perform nail services on a client with either a _____ or _____ of the skin.

34. List three infections of the skin that a nail technician cannot perform services if the client is infected.

    a. _____

    b. _____

    c. _____

35. **Matching.** Match the terms on the left with their correct descriptions on the right.

    _____ 1. leucoderma
    _____ 2. vitiligo
    _____ 3. lentigines
    _____ 4. chloasma
    _____ 5. athlete's foot
    _____ 6. albinism
    _____ 7. tan
    _____ 8. melanotic sarcoma
    _____ 9. keratoma
    _____ 10. mole
    _____ 11. ringworm of the hand
    _____ 12. nevus

    A. freckles
    B. general term for abnormal lack of pigmentation
    C. ultraviolet rays cause this skin darkening
    D. congenital absence of melanin
    E. skin cancer
    F. a callus
    G. a blackhead
    H. acquired form of leucoderma that affects skin or hair
    I. liver spots
    J. tinea pedis that is highly contagious
    K. a wart
    L. inflammatory skin condition with oozing blisters
    M. small brown spot on the skin
    N. red lesions occurring in patches or rings over the hands
    O. birthmark

MATCHING REVIEW

Insert the correct word listed in front of each definition below.

albininism
dermatology
dermis
epidermis
fissure
heat regulation

hypertropies
lesion
lymph
macule
melanin
nevus

scale
sebaceous
secretory
sensory
sudoriferous

57

36. _____ outer layer of the skin
37. _____ nerves of the sweat and oil glands
38. _____ study of healthy skin and skin disorders
39. _____ slightly yellow, watery fluid in the body
40. _____ also called sweat glands
41. _____ name of the skin coloring pigment
42. _____ examples are chapped hands or lips
43. _____ keeping the temperature at 98.6°F
44. _____ structural change in tissue caused by injury and disease
45. _____ also called the true skin or corium
46. _____ small, discolored spot or patch on the skin's surface
47. _____ also called oil gland
48. _____ a birthmark
49. _____ example is severe dandruff
50. _____ new growths

WORD REVIEW

If you do not know the meanings of the words listed below, look them up in the text.

absorption	external stimulus	respiration
adipose tissue	fissure	reticular layer
albinism	freckles	ringworm of the foot
arrector pili	fundus	ringworm of the hand
athlete's foot	heat regulation	scales
basal layer	herpes simplex	scar
blackhead	horny layer	scarf skin
blood	hypertropies	sebaceous glands
broken skin	infected skin	sebum
bulla	inflamed skin	secretory nerves
callus	keratoma	secretion
carbon dioxide	lentigines	sensory nerves
chloasma	lesions	stain
comedone	leucoderma	stratum corneum
complex sensations	lymph	stratum germinativum
corium	macule	stratum granulosum
corn	Malpighian layer	stratum lucidum
crust	melanin	stratum mucosum
cuticle	melanoma sarcoma	subcutaneous tissue
cutis	mole	sudoriferous glands
cyst	motor nerves	sweat glands
derma	nevus	sweat pore
dermatitis	nerve	tactile corpuscle
dermatology	nodule	tan
dermis	oil glands	tinea pedis
duct glands	oxygen	tumor
eczema	papillary layer	tubercle
elastic tissue	papule	ulcer
elasticity	protection	vesicle
epidermis	psoriasis	vitiligo
excoriation	pustule	wheals (hives)
excretion	raised skin	

Date _____

Rating _____

Text Pages 107-113

Client Consultation

COMPLETION

1. Define client consultation.
   _____

2. During the consultation, you will choose the _____ best suited for the client, and you will complete an evaluation about the _____ of the client's nails.

3. List four things that you would see if the client has a nail or skin disorder.
   a. _____
   b. _____
   c. _____
   d. _____

4. a. If you need to refer a client to a physician, you must act _____ and _____.
   b. To avoid causing unnecessary stress for your client, never attempt to _____ a problem or disorder.

5. If a client has an allergic reaction to a product, note on the client _____ which specific _____ caused the reaction.

6. The client has asked for a specific service. List two further questions you need to ask in relation to this service.
   a. _____
   b. _____

7. Does the client always know which service is the best one for him/her? Explain why or why not in detail.
   _____
   _____
   _____
   _____

8. Listed below are four different lifestyles or hobbies of people. Next to each one, list the types of nail and/or skin care these people may require.
   a. gardener: _____

59

b. guitar player: _____

   c. model: _____
   d. runner: _____

9. Performing a wrong service on a client could make that person unhappy and even cause _____ . If the client is not happy with the service, you will _____ a client.

10. a. After talking with the client about their needs, expectations, and health, you will either _____ the client's service choice or recommend _____ .

    b. List four things that you will explain at this time.
       1. _____
       2. _____
       3. _____
       4. _____

COMPLETION REVIEW

Insert the correct word listed in the sentences below.

card	disorder	product
client consultation	health	service
diagnose	open sores	tactfully

1. If you see inflammation, infection, redness, or _____ , it means that the client has a nail or skin _____ .

2. A meeting where you discuss the client's desires, needs, and nail health is called a/an _____ .

3. If a client has an allergic reaction to a product, note it on the client _____ .

4. During the consultation, you will choose the best suited _____ for the client.

5. If you need to refer a client to a physician, you must act responsibly and _____ .

WORD REVIEW

If you do not know the meanings of the words listed below, look them up in the text.

allergic reaction	disorders	job
appropriate	evaluation	lifestyle
client card	examine	nail health
client consultation	expectations	open skin
client desires	explain	recommend
client needs	hobbies	redness
decision	infection	result
diagnose	inflammation	safety

Part 3

BASIC PROCEDURES

- *CHAPTER 10* - Manicuring
- *CHAPTER 11* - Pedicuring

10

Date _____

Rating _____

Text Pages 116-143

Manicuring

EQUIPMENT

1. Manicuring equipment are _____ items and only when they wear out do they have to be _____ .

2. **Matching.** Match the terms on the left with their correct descriptions on the right.

   _____ 1. disinfection container
   _____ 2. supply tray
   _____ 3. client's cushion
   _____ 4. manicure table
   _____ 5. electric nail dryer
   _____ 6. cotton container
   _____ 7. fingerbowl

   A. used to trim away excess cuticle at the nail's base
   B. shaped for soaking the client's fingers
   C. shortens the nail drying time
   D. holds a disinfectant solution in which to immerse objects to be sanitized
   E. holds absorbent cotton or lint-free wipes
   F. also called a cuticle pusher
   G. most include a drawer to store sanitized implements
   H. adds shine to the nail plate
   I. holds polishes, polish removers, and creams
   J. can be either 8 by 12 inches or a folded towel

IMPLEMENTS

3. After using a manicuring implement on a client, the implement or tool must either be _____ or _____ .

4. What size are manicuring implements?
   _____

5. **Identification.** Using the letters **OS, MF, EB, CN, NB,** and **CB** (defined below), match the correct characteristics below with one manicuring implement.

   Key:
   OS = orangewood stick
   MF = metal nail file
   EB = emery board
   CN = cuticle nipper
   NB = nail brush
   CB = chamois buffer

Characteristics:

_____ 1. used to shape the free edge of hard nails

_____ 2. used to file soft or fragile nails

_____ 3. hold it so the blades face the cuticle

_____ 4. loosens the cuticle around the nail's base

_____ 5. adds shine to the nail

_____ 6. used to shape the free edge of sculptured nails

_____ 7. smooths out wavy ridges on the nails

_____ 8. remove bits of cuticle with warm soapy water

_____ 9. has a coarse and a fine side

_____ 10. used to clean under the free edge

_____ 11. used to cut or trim away excess cuticle

_____ 12. cleans the fingernails

6. a. A steel pusher is also called a/an _____ . It is used to push back excess cuticle _____ .

   b. The spoon end of a steel pusher is used to _____ and _____ cuticle.

7. Which implement is used to lift small bits of cuticle from the nail?
   _____

8. Name two implements that must be discarded if they are dropped on the floor.

   a. _____

   b. _____

9. How often must a metal nail file be disinfected?
   _____

10. a. List two types of chamois buffers.

    1. _____

    2. _____

    b. How often must a chamois be changed?
    _____

11. If your client's nails are very long, which implement can be used to shorten the filing time?
    _____

12. List the procedure for sanitizing implements.

    a. _____

    b. _____

    c. _____

    d. _____

    e. _____

63

13. Identify the parts, tools, and so forth on a manicuring table.

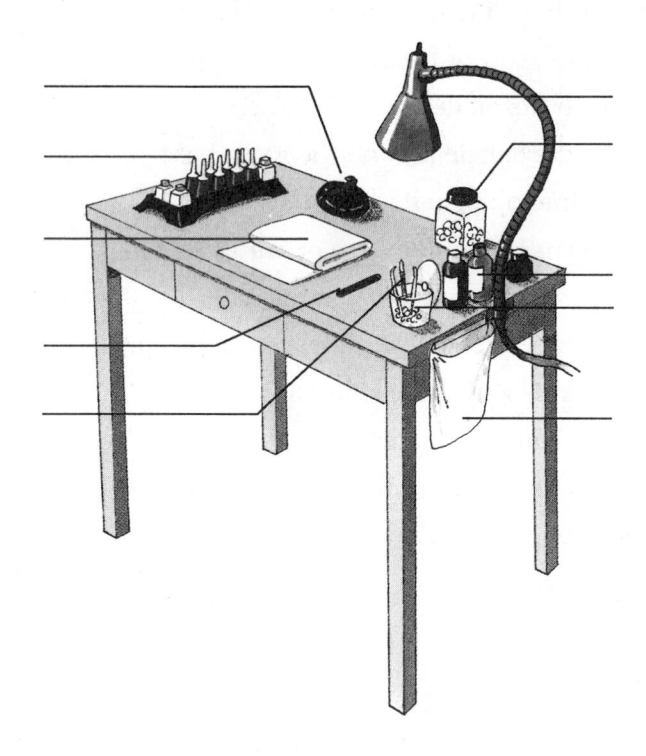

14. What is the usual soaking time for implements to be in a disinfection container?

15. Why is it a good idea to have two sets of metal implements?

MATERIALS

16. How often do manicuring materials need to be replaced? _____

17. **Matching.** Match the terms on the left with their correct descriptions on the right.

    _____ 1. plastic spatula   A. used to dry client's hand
    _____ 2. alum   B. shapes the nail's free edge
    _____ 3. plastic bags   C. used to stop bleeding
    _____ 4. towels   D. used to remove nail cosmetics from their containers
    _____ 5. cotton   E. used to soak client's hands
                                   F. holds discarded materials
                                   G. wrapped on the end of an orangewood stick

18. Why are styptic pencils not used in most states?

NAIL COSMETICS

19. **Matching.** Match the terms on the left with their correct descriptions on the right.

_____ 1. base coat
_____ 2. cuticle cream
_____ 3. cuticle oil
_____ 4. nail bleach
_____ 5. hand cream
_____ 6. antibacterial soap
_____ 7. top coat
_____ 8. colored polish, liquid enamel, or lacquer
_____ 9. nail strengthener/hardener
_____ 10. cuticle remover/solvent
_____ 11. nail whitener
_____ 12. polish remover
_____ 13. liquid nail dry
_____ 14. dry nail polish, or pumice powder

A. adds color to the nails; contains solution of nitrocellulose in a volatile solvent such as amyl acetate

B. used with warm water in a fingerbowl

C. keeps cuticle soft, contains vegetable oil, vitamin E, mineral oil, jojoba or palm nut oil

D. used to cut excess cuticle from the nails

E. applied under the free edge to make the nail appear white; contains zinc oxide or titanium dioxide

F. used with a chamois buffer to add shine; contains mild abrasives

G. removes nail polish; contains organic solvents and acetone

H. softens and smooths the hands; contains emollients and humectants, such as glycerin, cocoa butter, lecithin, and gums

I. contains 2-5% sodium or potassium hydroxide plus glycerin; makes cuticles easier to remove and minimizes clipping

J. promotes rapid polish drying; contains alcohol base

K. applied to the bare nail before polish; contains ethyl acetate, a solvent, isopropyl alcohol, butyl acetate, nitrocellulose, resin, and sometimes formaldehyde

L. used to sanitize the manicure table

M. lubricates and softens dry cuticles and brittle nails

N. bowl used to soak fingers

O. applied over colored polish to prevent chipping; contains nitrocellulose, toluene, a solvent, isopropyl alcohol, and polyester resins

P. removes yellow stains from the nail; contains hydrogen peroxide

Q. prevents splitting and peeling of the nail; can contain collagen, nylon fibers, or formaldehyde

20. List four forms of antibacterial soap.

a. _____
b. _____
c. _____
d. _____

21. a. List two ingredients found in polish remover.
    1. _____
    2. _____
    b. The type of polish remover to use on clients who have artificial nails is _____.

22. a. What ingredient is in nail bleach? _____
    b. If nail bleach gets on the skin, it may cause _____.

23. Why are nail white pencils not permitted in most states? _____

24. List two forms of dry nail polish.
    a. _____
    b. _____

25. Describe the purpose of a base coat. _____

26. List three types of nail strengtheners.
    a. _____
    b. _____
    c. _____

27. a. What is the base of a liquid nail dry? _____
    b. List two forms of liquid nail dry.
       1. _____
       2. _____

28. Which has a thicker consistency, hand cream or hand lotion? _____

PROCEDURE FOR BASIC TABLE SET-UP

29. When setting up for a manicure, the table should be wiped with a/an _____.

30. A client's cushion should be wrapped in a _____.

31. a. What goes into a disinfection container before putting your implements in it? _____
    b. Which manicuring implements are to be placed in the disinfection container? _____

32. If the manicurist is left-handed, on which side of the table is a plastic bag to be attached? _____

33. List five items that can be kept in the table drawer.

   a. _____
   b. _____
   c. _____
   d. _____
   e. _____

PREPARING CLIENT FOR A MANICURE

34. List four nail shapes.

   a. _____
   b. _____
   c. _____
   d. _____

35. Which nail shape is the most common choice for male client?
   _____

36. Which nail shape is well suited for thin hands?
   _____

37. Describe four considerations when deciding what nail shape is best for the client.

   a. _____
   b. _____
   c. _____
   d. _____

PROCEDURE FOR PLAIN WATER MANICURE

38. a. If the client is right-handed, with which of their hands do you begin a manicure?
   _____

   b. If the client is left-handed, with which of their hands do you begin a manicure?
   _____

   c. Why do you begin working on the hand that you do?
   _____

39. List the steps for a plain water manicure. Assume you are manicuring only one hand. Some steps are written for you.

   a. _Remove polish._____
   b. _Shape the nails._____
   c. _____
   d. _____
   e. _____
   f. _____
   g. _____

    h. _____
    i. _____
    j. ___Optional: Bleach nails._____
    k. _____
    l. _____
    m. _____
    n. _____
    o. _____
    p. _____
    q. ___Apply polish._____

40. To remove polish from the cuticle area, it may be necessary to put cotton on the tip of a/an _____ .

41. a. Nails are to be filed from corner to _____ .

    b. Explain why you shape the nails before soaking them.

    _____

    _____

42. If too much pressure is used when pushing the cuticle back at the base of the nail, it could cause damage to the _____ .

43. When nipping cuticles, be careful not to cut into the mantle as this will _____ .

44. What is the buffing pattern on the nails when using a chamois buffer?

    _____

45. a. List four coats of nail polish that are to be applied to the client's nails.

       1. _____
       2. _____
       3. _____
       4. _____

    b. Nail polish should be applied in how many strokes? _____

46. Polish corrector pens should not be used because they are _____ .

47. Identify the five types of polished nails:

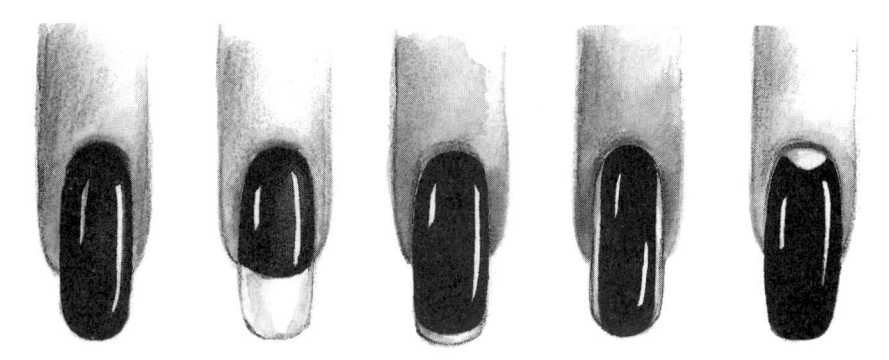

   _____ _____ _____ _____ _____

48. List five plain water manicure post-service procedures.

   a. _____
   b. _____
   c. _____
   d. _____
   e. _____

FRENCH MANICURE

49. List four steps of a French manicure.

   a. _____
   b. _____
   c. _____
   d. _____

RECONDITIONING MANICURE

50. List three items needed to perform a reconditioning manicure.

   a. _____
   b. _____
   c. _____

51. What is done in a reconditioning manicure that is not done in a plain water manicure?
   _____

ELECTRIC MANICURE

52. a. List four electric manicure attachments.

   1. _____
   2. _____
   3. _____
   4. _____

b. Using the four attachments you listed in question 52a, complete the following sentences. (Assume a plain manicure.)

1. A chamois buffer works like the _____ attachment.
2. An emery board is most like the _____ attachment.
3. A nail brush is like the _____ attachment.
4. A steel pusher is like the _____ attachment.

53. Using too much pressure on the nails with an electric manicure machine can cause the client to feel a/an _____ sensation.

PARAFFIN WAX

54. A paraffin treatment traps heat and moisture and _____ .
55. List two types of clients that will benefit from a paraffin treatment to the hands and feet.
    a. _____
    b. _____
56. How many times is the hand or foot dipped in paraffin?
    _____
57. How long is paraffin left on the hand or foot?
    _____

HAND AND ARM MASSAGE

58. List two things a massage does for the client.
    a. _____
    b. _____
59. In hand massage, the relaxer movement is also known as the _____ movement.
60. A light stroking massage movement that relaxes and soothes is called _____ .
61. A wringing movement on the arm is also known as a/an _____ type of massage movement.
62. Kneading the arm is also called the _____ movement. It is very stimulating and _____ blood flow.
63. Rotating the client's elbow is a type of massage movement known as _____ .

MATCHING REVIEW

Insert the correct word listed in front of each definition below.

alcohol
alum
approved hospital-grade
   disinfectant
base coat
chamois buffer
client's cushion
cuticle nipper

effleurage
electric manicure
electric nail dryer
emery board
fingerbowl
French manicure
hydrogen peroxide
left hand

nail bleach
nail strengthener
nail whitener
orangewood stick
petrissage
right hand
styptic pencil
supply tray

64. _____ has a coarse and a fine side
65. _____ on a right-handed person, begin with this
66. _____ a light stroking massage movement
67. _____ holds polishes, removers, and creams
68. _____ smooths out ridges and adds nail shine
69. _____ removes yellow stains from the nail
70. _____ shortens nail drying time
71. _____ prevents nail splitting and chipping
72. _____ used to cut away excess cuticle
73. _____ an ingredient in nail bleach
74. _____ either 8 by 12 inch or a folded towel
75. _____ applied to the bare nail before polish
76. _____ used to stop bleeding
77. _____ base ingredient of liquid nail dry
78. _____ used to clean under the free edge
79. _____ emery disk, cuticle pusher, cuticle brush, and buffer attachments
80. _____ an implement disinfectant
81. _____ a kneading massage movement
82. _____ shaped for soaking the client's fingers
83. _____ applied under the free edge to make the nail appear white

WORD REVIEW

If you do not know the meanings of the words listed below, look them up in the text.

abrasives	effleurage massage movement	hot oil heater
acetone	electric manicure	implements
adjustable lamp	electric nail dryer	joint massage movement
antibacterial soap	emery board	kneading massage movement
base coat	equipment	liquid enamel
bevel	fingerbowl	liquid nail dry
chamois buffer	fingernail clippers	manicure table
client chair	free edge polish application	materials
client's cushion	French manicure	metal nail file
colored polish	friction massage movement	nail bleach
cotton	full coverage polish	nail brush
cotton balls	application	nail cosmetics
cuticle cream	hairline tip polish application	nail lacquer
cuticle nipper	half moon or lunula polish	nail strengthener or hardener
cuticle oil	application	nail technician's chair or stool
cuticle solvent or remover	hand cream	nail whitener
disinfection container	hand lotion	non-acetone
disposable towels	hospital-grade disinfectant	orangewood stick
dry nail polish	hot oil	oval nail

71

paraffin
petrissage massage
  movement
plain water manicure
plastic bags
plastic spatula
pointed nails
polish remover

powdered alum
reconditioning manicure
rectangular or square nail
relaxer massage movement
round nail
sanitized cotton container
slim line or free-walls polish
  application

steel pusher
styptic powder
supply tray
terry towels
top coat
tweezers

11

Date _____

Rating _____

Text Pages 144-153

Pedicuring

INTRODUCTION

1. List four things included in a pedicure procedure.

   a. _____

   b. _____

   c. _____

   d. _____

2. Describe two improvements pedicures provide for a client.

   a. _____

   b. _____

3. a. What type of shoes should a client wear to the salon for their pedicure appointment?

   _____

   b. Why this type of shoe?

   _____

PEDICURE EQUIPMENT AND MATERIALS

4. **Matching.** Match the terms on the left with their correct descriptions on the right.

   _____ 1. foot bath   A. keeps toes apart
   _____ 2. toenail clippers   B. liquid soap with antibacterial agents
   _____ 3. pedicuring stool   C. should have an arm rest and be comfortable
   _____ 4. foot file   D. loosens the nail's cuticle
   _____ 5. foot powder   E. shortens toenails' length
   _____ 6. toe separators   F. disposable paper foot slippers
   _____ 7. pedicuring station   G. keeps feet dry after a pedicure
   _____ 8. foot lotion   H. filled with warm soapy water
   _____ 9. client's chair   I. includes two chairs and a foot rest
   _____ 10. antibacterial soap   J. used during a foot massage
                                     K. nail technician's low stool
                                     L. removes ingrown toenails
                                     M. removes dry skin or callus growth

73

PEDICURE PRE-SERVICE PROCEDURE

5. List three items that are part of a pedicure station set-up.
   a. _____
   b. _____
   c. _____

6. List two places where you should put towels in preparation for a pedicure.
   a. _____
   b. _____

7. Besides standard manicuring implements, list eight additional items for a pedicure.
   a. _____
   b. _____
   c. _____
   d. _____
   e. _____
   f. _____
   g. _____
   h. _____

8. Fill two basins with warm _____ . Then add to one basin _____, and add to the other basin _____.

9. What do you do if you notice an infection or inflammation on your client's feet?
   _____

PEDICURE PROCEDURE

10. List the steps for a pedicure procedure. Assume you are performing a pedicure on one foot. Some steps are written for you.
    a. __Remove shoes and socks.__
    b. _____
    c. _____
    d. _____
    e. _____
    f. _____
    g. _____
    h. _____
    i _____
    j. __Use foot file.__
    k. _____
    l. _____
    m. _____

n. _____Push cuticle back._____

o. _____

p. _____

q. _____

r. _____

s. _____

t. _____Powder feet._____

11. Client's feet should soak in a soap bath for at least _____ minutes.

12. In what shape should toenails be filed?
    _____

13. What can cause ingrown toenails?
    _____

14. List four coats of nail polish that are included in a pedicure service.

    a. _____
    b. _____
    c. _____
    d. _____

PEDICURE POST-SERVICE PROCEDURE

15. List six steps of a pedicure post-service procedure.

    a. _____
    b. _____
    c. _____
    d. _____
    e. _____
    f. _____

16. List three pedicure items that are to be wiped with hospital-grade disinfectant after using them.

    a. _____
    b. _____
    c. _____

FOOT MASSAGE

17. List three client medical conditions that could be dangerous to receive a foot massage.

    a. _____
    b. _____
    c. _____

18. The relaxing massage movement is called _____.
19. List four parts of the foot where this relaxing massage movement in question 18 is performed.
    a. _____
    b. _____
    c. _____
    d. _____
20. Deep rubbing movements, such as the thumb and fist twist compression, are also known as _____ massage movements.
21. What is another name for a kneading massage movement?
    _____
22. List two names used for a light tapping movement over the foot.
    a. _____
    b. _____
23. During a foot massage, a plantar's wart should not have _____ applied to that area.

MATCHING REVIEW

Insert the correct word/term listed in front of each definition below.

closed-toe	foot powder	petrissage
curved	friction	straight across
effleurage	open-toed	tapotement
foot bath	pedicure	toenail clippers
foot file	pedicuring stool	toe separators

24. _____ shortens the length of the toenails
25. _____ relaxing massage movement
26. _____ includes trimming, shaping, massage, and polishing the toenails
27. _____ removes dry skin or callus growth
28. _____ kneading massage movement
29. _____ shape toenails should be filed
30. _____ type of shoes client should wear for a pedicure appointment
31. _____ keeps toes apart during a pedicure
32. _____ a light, tapping massage movement
33. _____ filled with warm soapy water
34. _____ deep rubbing massage movements, such as thumb and fist twist compression
35. _____ keeps feet dry after a pedicure

WORD REVIEW

If you do not know the meanings of the words listed below, look them up in the text.

antibacterial soap	foot powder	petrissage
antiseptic antifungal foot spray	foot rest	plantar's wart
	friction	relaxer massage movement
callus	ingrown toenails	
client's chair	metatarsal scissors massage movement	tapotement
effleurage		thumb compression massage movement
fist twist massage movement	pedicure	
	pedicure slippers	toe separators
foot bath or basin	pedicure station	toenail clippers
foot file	pedicure stool	
foot lotion	percussion	

Part 4

THE ART OF NAIL TECHNOLOGY

- ◆ *CHAPTER 12* - Nail Tips
- ◆ *CHAPTER 13* - Nail Wraps
- ◆ *CHAPTER 14* - Acrylic Nails
- ◆ *CHAPTER 15* - Gels
- ◆ *CHAPTER 16* - The Creative Touch

12

Date _____

Rating _____

Text Pages 156-163

Nail Tips

INTRODUCTION

1. List three types of material out of which nail tips are made.

    a. _____

    b. _____

    c. _____

2. Name two other nail services with which nail tips are often combined.

    a. _____

    b. _____

3. A nail tip with no overlay is very _____. Consequently, it will not last long and is considered to be a/an _____ nail.

MATERIALS

4. What is a nail abrasive?

    _____

    _____

5. Define buffer block.

    _____

6. a. List two other names for nail adhesive.

    1. _____

    2. _____

    b. What is the purpose of this adhesive?

    _____

    c. Nail adhesive usually comes in a/an _____ with a pointed applicator _____ .

7. a. On a nail tip, its point of contact with the client's nail plate is called the tip's _____ .

    b. List two types of nail tip wells.

    1. _____

    2. _____

80

8. How much of a client's natural nail plate should a nail tip cover?
   _____

9. Define position stop.
   _____
   _____

NAIL TIP APPLICATION PRE-SERVICE

10. Besides the standard manicuring table, list four materials needed to apply nail tips.

    a. _____

    b. _____

    c. _____

    d. _____

11. With what type of soap should the client's hands be washed before the application of nail tips?
    _____

12. Label the half well, full well, and position stop on both pictures.

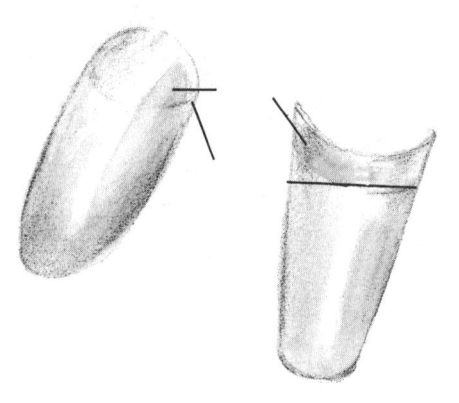

PROCEDURE

13. Under each of the following pictures, list the procedural step applying nail tips that is shown.

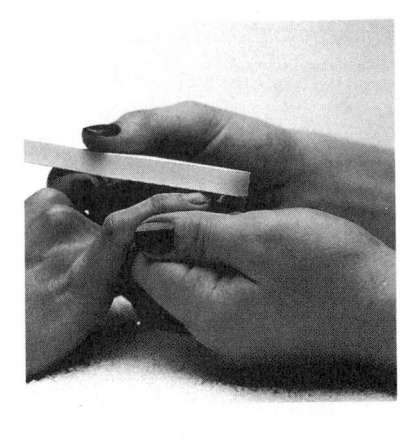

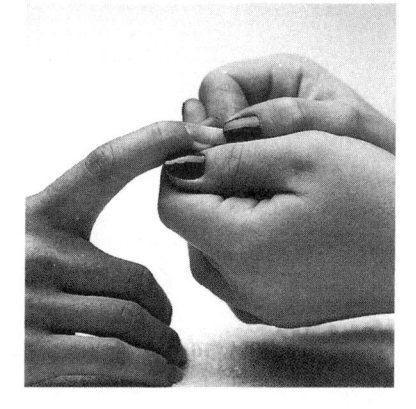

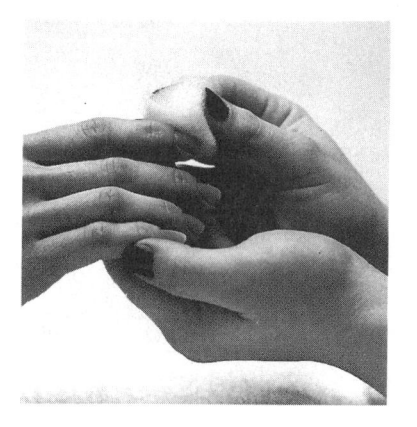

82

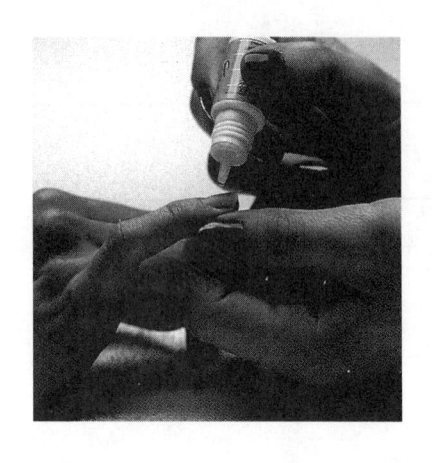

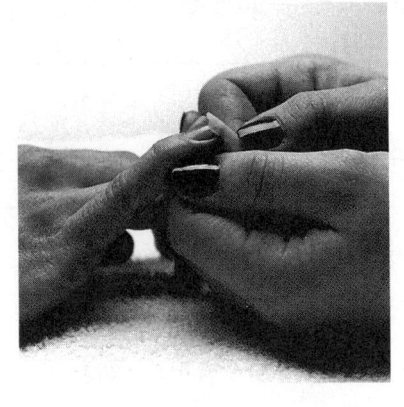

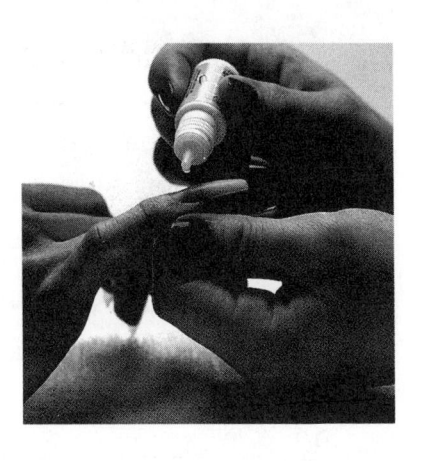

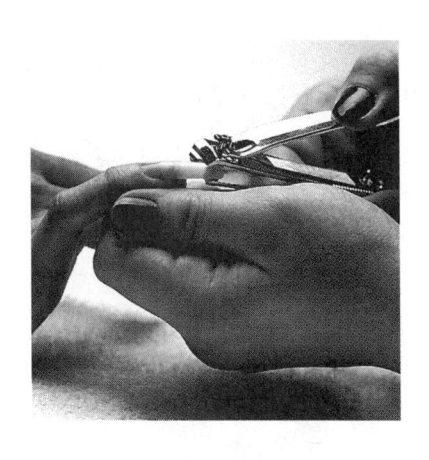

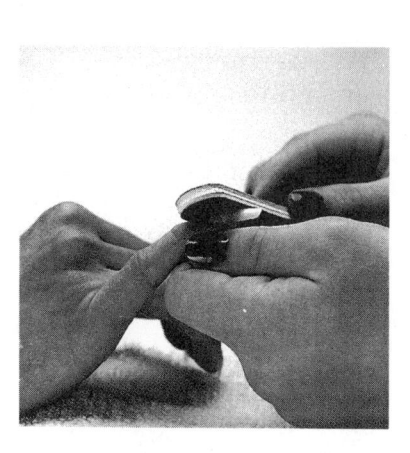

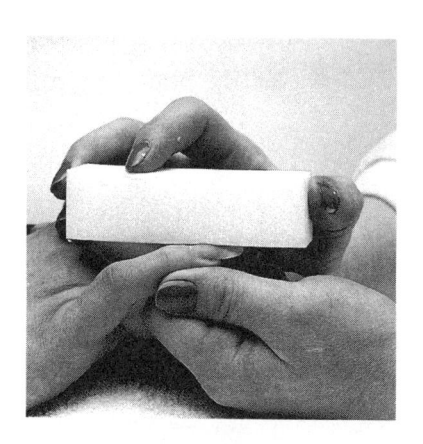

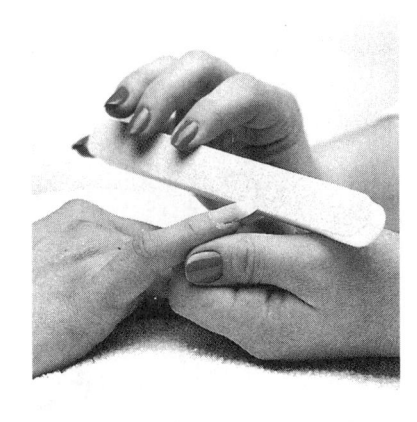

14. Besides sanitizing, list two other purposes of applying nail antiseptic.

    a. _____

    b. _____

15. If you accidentally touch the sanitized nails, you must _____ them.

16. Nail tips should cover the nail plate from sidewall to _____.

17. Why is a bead of adhesive applied to the seam?
    _____

18. a. Which implement is used to trim the nail to its desired length?
    _____

    b. How should the nail tip be cut?
    _____

    c. What happens if the tip is cut straight across?
    _____

19. a. When sanding the shine off of the nail tip, how should the file be held?
    _____

    b. Why?
    _____

20. Which implement is used to blend the tip into the nail plate?
    _____

21. Which implement is used to shape the end of the new, longer nail?
    _____

MAINTENANCE AND REMOVAL OF TIPS

22. List two reasons why clients with nail tips need regular manicures.

    a. _____

    b. _____

23. If a client has nail tips, what type of nail polish remover is used?
    _____

24. List two agents that will remove nail tips.

    a. _____

    b. _____

25. List the steps to remove nail tips.

    a. _____

    b. _____

    c. _____

    d. _____

    e. _____

    f. _____

MATCHING REVIEW

Insert the correct word/term listed in front of each definition below.

abrasive	disinfectant	non-acetone polish
acetone polish remover	emery board	remover
antiseptic	nail adhesive	position stop
buffer block	nail tips	well

26. _____ a lightweight rectangular item that is abrasive and used to buff the nails

27. _____ made out of plastic, nylon, or acetate

28. _____ sanitizes, removes natural oil, and dehydrates the nail

29. _____ on a nail tip, the point of contact with the client's nail plate

30. _____ also called glue or bonding agent

31. _____ used to remove polish and not remove nail tips

32. _____ a rough surface used to shape or smooth the nail and remove the shine

33. _____ point where the nail plate meets the tip before it is glued to the nail

WORD REVIEW

If you do not know the meaning of the words listed below, look them up in the text.

abrasive	glue remover	plastic
acetate	nail adhesive	position stop
acetone polish remover	nail antiseptic	seam
bonding agent	nail tip/s	sidewall
buffer block	non-acetone polish remover	stress point
full well	nylon	well
glue	partial/half well	

13

Date _____

Rating _____

Text Pages 164-174

Nail Wraps

INTRODUCTION

1. Define nail wraps.

   _____

   _____

2. List two purposes of nail wraps.

   a. _____

   b. _____

3. Where are pre-cut overlays attached to the nail?

   _____

4. a. List three types of fabric wraps.

   1. _____

   2. _____

   3. _____

   b. Which of the three fabric wraps is opaque, thereby needing colored polish to cover it after it is applied?

   _____

   c. Which of the three fabric wraps is transparent and may or may not need colored polish?

   _____

   d. Which of the three fabric wraps has a loose weave that makes it easy for the adhesive to protect?

   _____

5. a. List two chemicals that dissovle paper wraps.

   1. _____

   2. _____

   b. How often do paper wraps have to be replaced?

   _____

PROCEDURE FOR APPLYING FABRIC WRAPS

6. Besides your basic manicure table set-up, list six other materials you will need for applying fabric wraps.

   a. _____
   b. _____
   c. _____
   d. _____
   e. _____
   f. _____

7. Write in the steps of a nail wrap procedure. Some of them are completed for you.

   a. _____Remove old polish._____
   b. _____
   c. _____
   d. _____
   e. _____
   f. _____
   g. _____Cut fabric._____
   h. _____
   i. _____
   j. _____
   k. _____
   l. _____
   m. _____Apply second coat of adhesive._____
   n. _____
   o. _____
   p. _____
   q. _____
   r. _____Apply polish._____

8. How far from the sidewalls and free edge should the fabric be trimmed?
   _____

9. What sensation will the client feel if you get some adhesive dryer on the skin during the application?
   _____

10. How do you apply the second coat of adhesive in order to prevent lifting?
    _____
    _____
    _____

11. a. What two items do you use to buff the nails after the wraps are on?

    1. _____
    2. _____

    b. Why do you buff the wrap(s)?
    _____

    c. What can happen if you buff too much or too hard?
    _____

12. How do you remove traces of oil from the nail?
    _____

NAIL WRAP POST-SERVICE PROCEDURE

13. How do you clean clogged extender tips?
    _____
    _____

14. In most states, implements need to be sanitized for _____ minutes before they can be used on the next client.

FABRIC WRAP MAINTENANCE

15. a. Do you apply additional fabric to your client's wrap(s) two weeks after the wrap(s) were applied?
    _____

    b. In a two-week fabric wrap maintenance application, what do you apply to the new growth first, and then to the entire nail?
    _____

16. a. Do you apply additional fabric to your client's wrap(s) four weeks after the wrap(s) were applied?
    _____

    b. How is the procedure in question 16a above applied?
    _____
    _____

FABRIC WRAP REPAIR

17. List two reasons for fabric wrap repair.

    a. _____
    b. _____

18. Define repair patch.
    _____
    _____

19. How do you apply a repair patch?
   _____
   _____

FABRIC WRAP REMOVAL

20. Using the letters a, b, c, d, and e, put the following steps in correct sequential order to remove fabric wraps.

    _____ buff nails

    _____ soak nails

    _____ condition cuticles

    _____ complete nail wrap pre-service preparation

    _____ slide off softened wraps

21. To remove nail wraps, what do you soak the nails in?
    _____

22. a. When buffing the nails, what side of the block buffer is used?
       _____

    b. What does buffing remove?
       _____

PAPER WRAPS

23. What is the name of the thin paper used for paper wraps?
    _____

24. How long do paper wraps last?
    _____

25. Concerning paper wraps, what specifically does nail polish remover dissolve?
    _____

26. Why aren't paper wraps recommended for extra long nails?
    _____

MATERIALS

27. List three materials needed for paper wraps.

    a. _____

    b. _____

    c. _____

28. Mending liquid is applied with a/an _____.

PAPER WRAP APPLICATION PROCEDURE

29. Below each diagram, list the correct procedural step for a paper wrap.

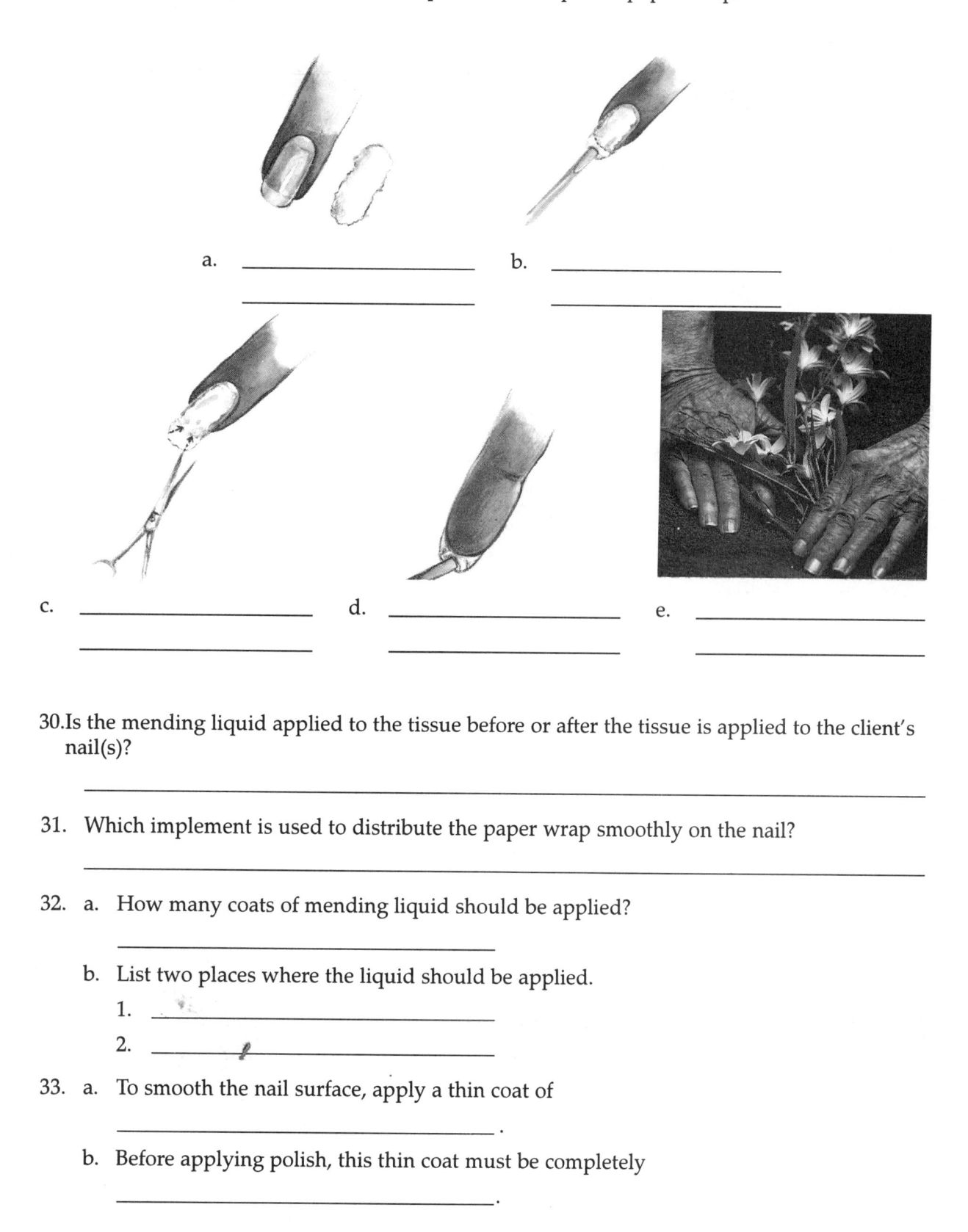

a. _____   b. _____

c. _____   d. _____   e. _____

30. Is the mending liquid applied to the tissue before or after the tissue is applied to the client's nail(s)?
_____

31. Which implement is used to distribute the paper wrap smoothly on the nail?
_____

32. a. How many coats of mending liquid should be applied?
    _____

   b. List two places where the liquid should be applied.
      1. _____
      2. _____

33. a. To smooth the nail surface, apply a thin coat of
      _____ .

   b. Before applying polish, this thin coat must be completely
      _____ .

89

LIQUID NAIL WRAP

34. Define liquid nail wrap.

   _____
   _____

35. How is liquid nail wrap applied?

   _____

36. Explain the difference between liquid nail wrap and nail hardener.

   _____

MATCHING REVIEW

Insert the correct word/term listed in front of each definition below.

acetone	fiberglass	nail adhesive
block buffer	heat	nail wraps
cold	linen	paper wraps
fabric wraps	mending tissue	repair patch

37. _____ are temporary and must be replaced when polish is removed.

38. _____ three types are silk, linen, and fiberglass

39. _____ piece of fabric cut so that it completely covers the crack or break in the nail

40. _____ is opaque so it needs colored polish when it is on the nails

41. _____ sensation the client feels is adhesive dryer gets on their skin

42. _____ thin paper used for paper wraps

43. _____ used to smooth out rough areas in the fabric

44. _____ has a loose weave so that adhesive penetrates easily

45. _____ used to remove nail wraps

46. _____ nail-size pieces of cloth or paper that are bonded to the front of the nail plate with nail adhesive

WORD REVIEW

If you do not know the meanings of the words isted below, look them up in the text.

abrasive	mending tissue	repair patch
adhesive dryer	nail adhesive/glue	ridge filler
adhesive extender tip	nail antiseptic	silk
fabric	nail block buffer	small scissors
fiberglass	nail wraps	stress strip
linen	opaque	transparent
liquid nail wrap	overlays	
mending liquid	paper wraps	

14

Date _____

Rating _____

Text Pages 175-191

Acrylic Nails

INTRODUCTION

1. Another name for sculptured nails is _____ nails.

2. a. List two products from which sculptured nails are made.

   1. _____
   2. _____

   b. These two products form a soft _____ that can easily be molded into a nail _____.

3. List three nail items over which sculptured nails can be applied.

   a. _____
   b. _____
   c. _____

4. Give three reasons or purposes of having sculptured nails applied to nails.

   a. _____
   b. _____
   c. _____

5. An acrylic nail should conform to the shape of the client's fingers and _____.

6. a. List three ingredients of acrylic nails.

   1. _____
   2. _____
   3. _____

   b. Of the three ingredients in question 6 above:

   1. acrylic liquid is a type of _____.
   2. a finished acrylic nail is a _____.
   3. an ingredient that speeds up the hardening process is a _____.

   c. Another word for the hardening process is _____.

91

7. Name two items that combine to make up the powder into which you dip your brush.

   a. _____

   b. _____

8. Define polymerization.
   _____

9. a. List two methods of applying acrylic nails.

   1. _____

   2. _____

   b. Which of the two methods looks like a French manicure and need no polish?
   _____

   c. Which of the two methods creates a chalky white nail that needs colored polish or a clear, shiny coating that allows the natural nail to show through?
   _____

MATERIALS

10. Besides basic manicuring tools or equipment, list ten other items needed to apply sculptured nails.

    a. _____
    b. _____
    c. _____
    d. _____
    e. _____
    f. _____
    g. _____
    h. _____
    i. _____
    j. _____

11. a. Why is primer used?
    _____

    b. List two types of primer.

    1. _____

    2. _____

    c. Which type of primer is easier to use safely?
    _____

    d. Which type of primer can cause serious damage to the skin and eyes?
    _____

    e. List two safety items you should wear when applying primer.

    1. _____

    2. _____

    f.   What should you do if you spill primer on your clothing?

   _____

12. a.   The two types of nail forms are reusable and _____ .

    b.   Which type of nail form in question 12a above has an adhesive backing to hold it in place?

          _____

    c.   Name three kinds of material out of which **reusable** nail forms are made.

        1. _____

        2. _____

        3. _____

13. What is used to apply and shape soft balls of acrylic on the nail?

_____

PROCEDURE

14. Which is applied first, primer or nail antiseptic?

    _____

15. What color is the primer when it dries on the nail?

    _____

16. When positioning the nail form, the client's free edge is to be _____ the form.

17. Place the number 1, 2, 3, 4, 5, or 6 beside each diagram to show correct procedural order.

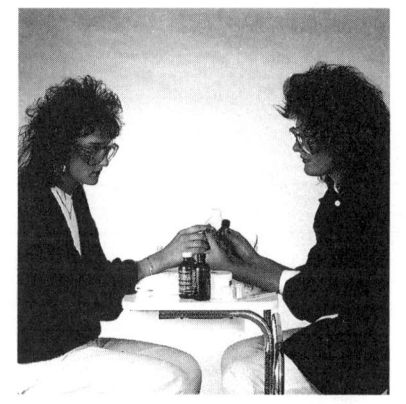

_____ Always wear safety glasses when applying primer.

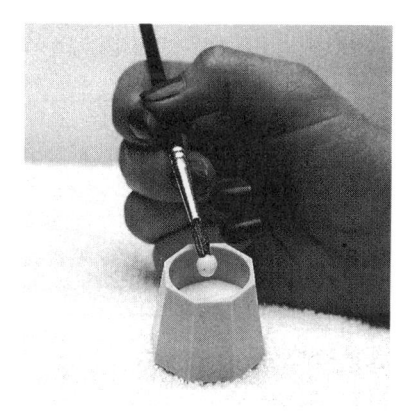

_____ Form ball of acrylic.

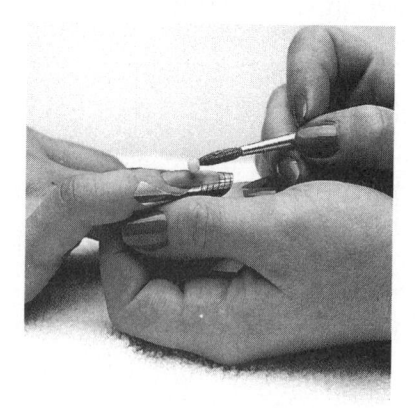

_____ Place ball on natural nail.

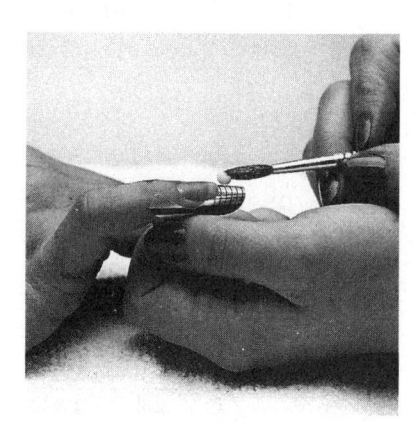

_____ Place ball of acrylic on nail form.

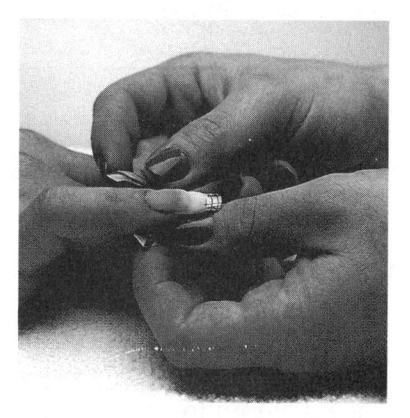

_____ Remove forms

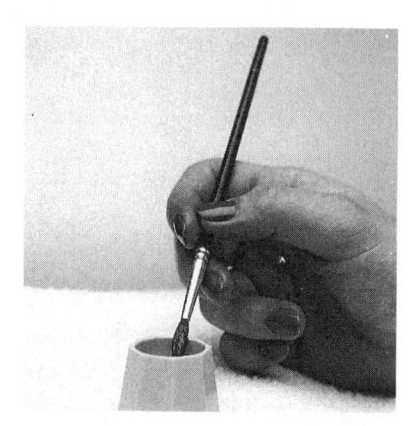

_____ Dip brush into acrylic liquid.

18. a. Where is the first ball of acrylic placed?

   _____

   b. Where is the second acrylic ball placed?

   _____

19. What part of the sable brush is used to dab and press the acrylic?

   _____

20. Define acrylic beads.

   _____

   _____

21. a. How do you know when the acrylic nail is dry?

   _____

   b. When the nails are dry, what is the next step you do?

   _____

22. Assume that you have just removed the nail forms. Use the letters a, b, c, d, e, f, and g to show the correct order of the following steps.

   _____ clean nails

   _____ buff the acrylic nail with block buffer

94

_____ apply polish

_____ clean up your work area or table

_____ apply oil to cuticles

_____ shape the free edge of the acrylic nail with a coarse or medium abrasive

_____ apply cream and perform massage

ACRYLIC APPLICATION POST-SERVICE PROCEDURE

23. After the service, what do you do with acrylic liquid and powder left in the small containers?
    _____

24. Name two items that can be used to clean your sable brush.

    a. _____

    b. _____

25. Bristles should not be pulled out of a brush because _____ .

26. a. How should acrylic powders be stored?
    _____

    b. What two items are to be stored in cool, dark places?

       1. _____

       2. _____

    c. Acrylic nail products should not be stored near _____ .

ACRYLIC APPLICATION OVER TIPS OR NATURAL NAILS

27. **Matching.** The left column contains the correct acrylic nail procedure. Match these items with their specific descriptions, directions, or characteristics listed in the right column. The first one is done for you.

_(E)_	1. push cuticle back	A.	wear plastic gloves and safety glasses
_____	2. buff to remove shine	B.	dip briefly in antibacterial soap and water
_____	3. clean nails	C.	place on nail plate
_____	4. apply nail antiseptic	D.	rub into cuticles and surrounding skin
_____	5. apply tips	E.	use a light touch because the cuticle is dry
_____	6. apply primer	F.	pick up medium, dry ball
_____	7. prepare liquid and powder	G.	base coat, polish, top coat
_____	8. dip brush into liquid and powder	H.	attach plastic nails to client's natural nails
_____	9. place first ball	I.	small wet balls used to smooth entire acrylic surface.
_____	10. place second ball	J.	use medium/fine file to remove natural oil(s)
_____	11. apply acrylic beads	K.	use block buffer to smooth entire acrylic surface
_____	12. shape nail		

95

_____ 13. buff nail
_____ 14. apply cuticle oil
_____ 15. massage hands and arms
_____ 16. apply polish

L. use in small, separate containers
M. place on nail's free edge
N. use orangewood stick, cotton, or spray to prevent bacteria growth
O. use coarse abrasive on the free edge
P. use hand cream or lotion

ACRYLIC NAIL APPLICATION OVER BITTEN NAILS

28. Explain the difference in applying acrylics over bitten nails compared with applying acrylics over forms.

   _____
   _____

29. Where is the first ball of acrylic applied?

   _____

30. What is done after this first ball of acrylic has been shaped and dried?

   _____

31. Explain where a nail form is placed.

   _____

32. Once the nail forms are on, the procedure follows the same steps as for acrylic nails over _____ .

33. Explain what procedural step is occurring in each of the following diagrams.

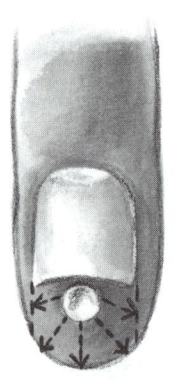

   _____

   _____

96

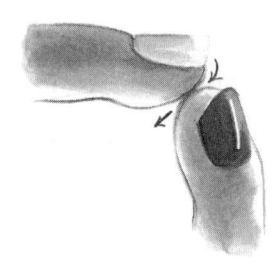

ACRYLIC NAIL MAINTENANCE

34. List two things that regular maintenance of acrylic nails helps to prevent.

    a. _____

    b. _____

35. Explain what can happen if a client does not maintain acrylic nails.

    _____

    _____

ACRYLIC NAIL MAINTENANCE

36. Define acrylic rebalancing.

    _____

37. How often should acrylic nails be rebalanced?

    _____

38. List the missing steps in the following procedure for acrylic nail rebalancing.

    a. ___Remove old polish._____

    b. _____

    c. ___Refine, then buff the nail._____

    d. _____

    e. ___Clean the nail._____

    f. _____

    g. ___Buff the nail to remove shine or natural oil._____

    h. _____

    i. ___Apply primer._____

    j. _____

    k. ___Place and shape balls of acrylic._____

    l. ___Shape, then buff the nail._____

    m. _____

    n. ___Apply hand cream and massage hand and arm._____

    o. _____

    p. ___Apply polish._____

97

39. a. Should a nipper be used to cut away loose acrylic?
       _____

    b. Why or why not?
       _____

40. Explain what should be done if a client has excessive, or a lot of acrylic lifting.
    _____
    _____

ACRYLIC CRACK REPAIR

41. Define acrylic crack repair.
    _____
    _____

42. List two ways the cracked acrylic can be filed.
    a. _____
    b. _____

43. In performing an acrylic crack repair, when would a nail form be used?
    _____

44. Where are the first balls, or beads, of acrylic placed or applied?
    _____

ACRYLIC REMOVAL

45. List five steps to removing acrylics.
    a. _____
    b. _____
    c. _____
    d. _____
    e. _____

46. The client's fingertips should be soaked for _____ minutes or as long as needed to _____ the acrylic product. For acrylic removal, refer to your _____ directions.

ODORLESS ACRYLICS

47. Are odorless acrylics completely odorless?
    _____

48. a. Which type of acrylic is wetter, traditional or odorless acrylic?
       _____

    b. Shaping odorless acrylics can be done at a _____ pace than traditional acrylics.

98

49. Explain the self-leveling characteristics of odorless acrylics.
   _____

50. a. What is the surface like when odorless acrylics are dry?
   _____

   b. What happens to this residue as you refine the nails?
   _____

51. Explain why traditional and odorless acrylic products cannot be mixed together.
   _____

MATCHING REVIEW

Insert the correct word listed in front of each definition below.

acrylic	monomer	rebalancing
catalyst	non-etching	reusable forms
curing	polymer	sable brush
disposable forms	polymerization	
etching	primer	

52. _____ ingredient that speeds up the hardening process
53. _____ type of primer than can damage the skin and eyes
54. _____ process of forming the nail
55. _____ another name for sculptured nails
56. _____ addition of acrylic to the new growth area of the nails
57. _____ made out of aluminum, Teflon, or plastic
58. _____ example is acrylic liquid
59. _____ type of primer that can be used safely
60. _____ another name for the hardening process
61. _____ used to apply and shape soft balls of acrylic on the nail

WORD REVIEW

If you do not know the meanings of the words listed below, look them up in the text.

acetone	crack repair	polymer
acrylic beads	curing	polymerization
acrylic liquid	etching	primer
acrylic maintenance	monomer	rebalancing
acrylic nails	nail antiseptic	sable brush
acrylic powder	nail forms	safety glasses
antibacterial soap	non-acetone	sculptured nails
ball of acrylic	non-etching	self-leveling
bitten nails	odorless acrylics	two-color method
catalyst	one-color method	

15

Date _____

Rating _____

Text Pages 192-200

Gels

INTRODUCTION

1. List two types of gel nails.

    a. _____

    b. _____

2. Which type of gel is hardened by a special light source?

    _____

3. Name two sources of this special light.

    a. _____

    b. _____

4. Explain how no-light gels harden.

    _____

5. **True/False.** The following statements concern the color of gel nails. Mark the true statements with a **T** and the false statements with an **F**.

    _____ 1. Gels are available in colors that do not need polish.

    _____ 2. Colored gels are not a base for nail art.

    _____ 3. Polish will permanently change the color of gel.

    _____ 4. Gel nails must always be polished.

    _____ 5. Polish may be worn over colored gels.

    _____ 6. Colored gels are a great base for nail. art.

    _____ 7. Gels stay the same color until the gel is removed.

    _____ 8. Polish cannot be worn over gels.

MATERIALS NEEDED FOR LIGHT-GEL APPLICATION

6. List eight items needed for gel nails.

    a. _____   e. _____

    b. _____   f. _____

    c. _____   g. _____

    d. _____   h. _____

7. What is a curing light?

    _____

    _____

GEL APPLICATION PRE-SERVICE PROCEDURE

8. Before applying gels, the client's hands are to be washed with _____ soap.

LIGHT-CURED GEL PROCEDURE

9. **Directions.** Using the list on top, fill in the bottom list with the application for light-cured gels in their correct procedural steps.

   Clean nails.
   Push back cuticles.
   Apply second coat of gel.
   Apply tips.
   Cure first coat of gel.

   Apply cream and perform massage.
   Remove polish.
   Clean nails.
   Apply primer.
   Buff nails to remove shine.

   Apply cuticle oil.
   Apply polish.
   Cure second coat of gel.
   Apply nail antiseptic.
   Clean nails.
   Apply first coat of gel.

   a. _____
   b. _____
   c. _____
   d. _____
   e. _____
   f. _____
   g. _____
   h. _____
   i. _____
   j. _____
   k. _____
   l. _____
   m. _____
   n. _____
   o. _____
   p. _____

10. Gel is applied to the nail by brushing it on in a thin, _____ layer.

11. The gel will lift if it is brushed onto the _____ .

12. How do you know the amount of minutes needed under the gel light?
    _____

13. Which type of gel light/lamp can cause damage to the eyes and skin?
    _____

GEL APPLICATION POST-SERVICE PROCEDURE

14. List five things you are to do after completing a gel nail application.

    a. _____
    b. _____
    c. _____

d. _____

e. _____

15. In most states, sanitizing implements means that before using them on the next client, items are to be sanitized for _____ minutes.

LIGHT-CURED GEL APPLIED ON FORMS

16. Fill in the missing procedural steps for light-cured gels applied onto nail forms.

    a. __Apply nail forms._____

    b. _____

    c. __Cure the gel._____

    d. _____

    e. __Cure the gel._____

    f. _____

    g. __Cure the gel._____

    h. __Remove the forms._____

    i. _____

    j. __Apply gel to the entire nail without the form._____

    k. _____

    l. __Remove residue._____

    m. _____

    n. __Apply hand cream and perform massage._____

    o. _____

    p. __Apply polish._____

17. What is meant by remove residue?

    _____

    _____

18. Below each figure, list the procedural step that is shown.

    a. _____

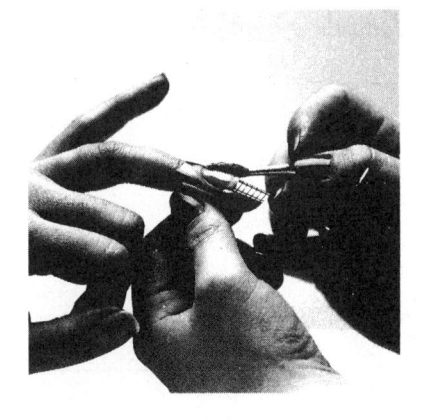

102

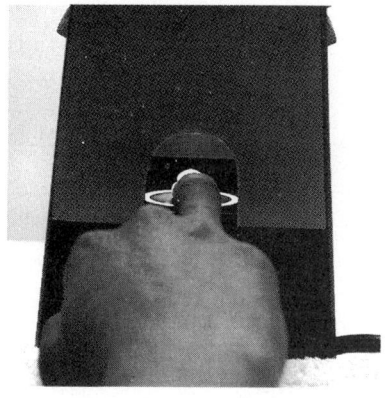

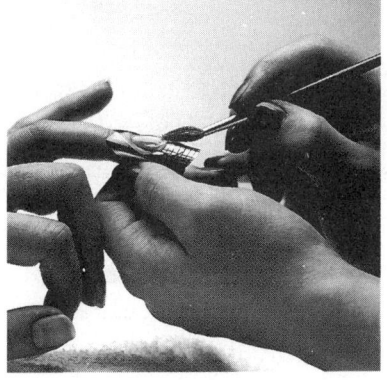

b. _____   c. _____

PROCEDURE FOR NO-LIGHT GEL APPLICATION

19. List two no-light curing agents.

    a. _____

    b. _____

20. Because curing agents vary for no-light gels, it is essential that you read and follow the _____ directions.

21. a. If the gels are water cured, the temperature of the water should be _____ .

    b. Depending on the manufacturer's directions, water cured gels should be immersed for _____ to _____ minutes.

22. a. What is another name for spray or brush gel activator?
    _____

    b. A spray gel activator should be held _____ inches away from the client's _____ . This is to reduce the chance of the client experiencing a _____ reaction from the activator.

GEL MAINTENANCE

23. How often should gel nails be maintained?
    _____

24. Before applying new gel, the old gel must be buffed. You buff until
    _____

25. a. Explain how the file should be held for buffing.
    _____

    b. Why should you hold the file in this way?
    _____

26. After the buffing is completed, what procedure is followed to maintain the gels?
    _____

GEL REMOVAL

27. List two products that will remove gels.

    a. _____

    b. _____

28. What type of bowl should be used to remove gels?

    _____

29. For a few minutes, the client's nails should be _____ in one of two products. Then the softened gel should be gently pushed off using a/an _____.

MATCHING REVIEW

Insert the correct word listed in front of each definition below.

acetone   curing light   ultraviolet
adhesive dryer   light-cured   safety glasses
antibacterial   lukewarm   steel pusher
apron   orangewood stick
cold   regrowth ledge

30. _____ nails hardened by a special light source
31. _____ a product that will remove gel nails
32. _____ box with ultraviolet or halogen bulb to cure or harden gel nails
33. _____ another name for spray or brush gel activator
34. _____ type of soap used to wash client's hands
35. _____ type of light that can harm the eyes and skin
36. _____ temperature of water to cure gels
37. _____ area to be removed in gel maintenance
38. _____ used to gently slide off softened gel tip
39. _____ wear when applying primer

WORD REVIEW

If you do not know the meanings of the words listed below, look them up in the text.

adhesive dryer   gels   regrowth ledge
brush gel activator   halogen light   spray gel activator
cure   light-cured gels   ultraviolet light
curing light   no-light gels

16

Date _____

Rating _____

Text Pages 201-218

The Creative Touch

CREATING NAIL ART

1. List four types/tools of nail art.

   a. _____

   b. _____

   c. _____

   d. _____

2. To interest clients in nail art, you might want to wear artistic designs on _____ nails.

3. **Identification.** Using the letters **G, T, F,** and **A** (defined below), match the correct characteristics listed below with one form of nail art.

   Key:

   G = gems

   T = striping tape

   F = foil

   A = applies to all three forms (gems, tape, and foil)

   Characteristics:

   _____ 1. comes in sheets and is applied to tacky top coat

   _____ 2. to remove, use acetone

   _____ 3. gives sparkle and texture and is applied to tacky top coat

   _____ 4. comes in rolls

   _____ 5. can be reused if the silver backing is in place

   _____ 6. is made of very fragile leafing

   _____ 7. to maintain, reapply top coat every 3-4 days

   _____ 8. applied to a dry, polished nail

4. The technique of airbrushing two or more colors on the nail at the same time is called the _____ or _____ .

5. How does an airbrush work?

   _____

6. List three ways in which airbrushes differ.
   a. _____
   b. _____
   c. _____

7. When learning airbrush techniques, practice them on what four surfaces?
   a. _____
   b. _____
   c. _____
   d. _____

8. Write in the steps of an airbrushing procedure. Some of them are completed for you.
   a. _____Complete the nail service and have client pay bill._____
   b. _____
   c. _____
   d. _____Airbrush nails._____
   e. _____
   f. _____
   g. _____
   h. _____Cleanse the fingers or toes._____
   i. _____

9. List two popular airbrush techniques.
   a. _____
   b. _____

MATCHING REVIEW

Insert the correct word listed in front of each definition below.

absorbent paper	foil	steel pusher
acetone	gems	striping tape
airbrush	mask knife	tweezers
color fade	nail art	
design tool	paint bonder	

10. _____ made of very fragile leafing
11. _____ includes gems, foils, tape and airbrushing
12. _____ a compressor that pushes air through a brush
13. _____ used to place gems on nails
14. _____ comes in rolls
15. _____ popular airbrush
16. _____ good for practicing airbrushing
17. _____ applied over dry airbrushed nails

18. _____ used to draw with airbrush
19. _____ best for removing airbrushed nail color

WORD REVIEW

If you do not know the meanings of the words listed below, look them up in the text.

air hose	French manicure	overspray
air source	gems	paint bonder
airbrush	gravity-fed	pearlescent paint
color blend	internal mix	reservoir
color fade	mask knife	striping tape
compressor	mask paper	stencil
design tool	nail art	
foil	nail glaze	

Part 5

THE BUSINESS OF NAIL TECHNOLOGY

◆ *CHAPTER 17* - Salon Business

◆ *CHAPTER 18* - Selling Nail Products and Services

17

Date _____

Rating _____

Text Pages 220-227

Salon Business

INTRODUCTION

1. To be financially successful, a nail technician must not only know how to perform nail services well, but must also be a good _____ person.

2. List six expenses a salon owner pays.

   a. _____
   b. _____
   c. _____
   d. _____
   e. _____
   f. _____

YOUR WORKING ENVIRONMENT

1. **Identification.** Using the letters **FS** and **NO** (defined below), match the correct characteristics listed below with one type of salon.

   Key:
   FS = full-service salon
   NO = nails-only salon

   Characteristics:

   _____ 1. often employ only one nail technician
   _____ 2. you will work with other nail technicians
   _____ 3. you automatically get all of the nail care business
   _____ 4. clients may take nail care more seriously
   _____ 5. clients conveniently get their nails and hair done at the same time

4. Briefly list eleven items you should consider when deciding on a salon that is right for you.

   a. _____
   b. _____
   c. _____
   d. _____
   _____

110

e. _____
f. _____
g. _____
h. _____
i. _____
j. _____
k. _____
_____

KEEPING GOOD PERSONAL RECORDS

5. List four business/financial items you should save.

   a. _____
   b. _____
   c. _____
   d. _____

6. a. Define income.
   _____

   b. List four sources of salon income.

      1. _____
      2. _____
      3. _____
      4. _____

7. a. Define expenses.
   _____

   b. List six personal salon expenses.

      1. _____
      2. _____
      3. _____
      4. _____
      5. _____
      6. _____

UNDERSTANDING SALON BUSINESS RECORDS

8. Explain four reasons for keeping accurate business records.

   a. _____
   b. _____
   c. _____
   d. _____
   _____

9. **Identification.** Using the numbers **1** and **7** (defined below), match the correct type of business record with the number of years it should be kept.

   Key:
   1 = business records should be kept for at least 1 year
   7 = business records should be kept for at least 7 years

   Business Records:

   _____ 1. monthly and yearly records
   _____ 2. daily sales slips
   _____ 3. cancelled checks
   _____ 4. inventory records
   _____ 5. appointment book
   _____ 6. payroll book
   _____ 7. petty cash book
   _____ 8. service records

10. **Matching.** Match the terms of the left with their correct descriptions on the right.

    _____ 1. inventory
    _____ 2. retail supplies
    _____ 3. changes in demands for services
    _____ 4. personal appointment records
    _____ 5. consumption supplies
    _____ 6. profit and loss comparisons
    _____ 7. service record
    _____ 8. net income

    A. over a period of time to see the slow versus busiest months
    B. supplies sold
    C. tells you who your next client is and what service you are to perform
    D. your income minus expenses
    E. the money you make
    F. if not successful, you may decide to cut that service from your business
    G. being a salaried employee versus an independent contractor
    H. with accurate records, you can cut costs by keeping appropriate stock levels and detect theft loss
    I. supplies used in the business
    J. the money you spend
    K. a list of treatments given and merchandise sold to each client

BOOKING APPOINTMENTS

11. List six items that are needed to supply the appointment desk/book.

    a. _____
    b. _____
    c. _____
    d. _____

e. _____

f. _____

12. a. When acknowledging your client's presence at the counter, try not to keep them _____ .

b. When answering the phone, identify both yourself and the salon by _____ .

c. Let clients know you are _____ to talk with them.

d. Don't mumble or shout, but speak _____ to the client.

e. If you have appointments made in advance, it is a good practice to _____ your clients the night before the appointment to _____ them and confirm the _____ .

f. At the end of their appointment, always ask your clients if they wish to _____ .

13. What five items are to be written in the appointment book when a client makes an appointment?

a. _____
b. _____
c. _____
d. _____
e. _____

ADVERTISING YOURSELF

14. a. List three items that are to be included on a list of every service you offer.

1. _____
2. _____
3. _____

b. In what two places should you distribute this service list?

1. _____
2. _____

COLLECTING PAYMENT FOR SERVICES

15. In some salons, payments for services are collected by the _____ , while in other salons it is collected by the _____ .

16. List four items to be included on a client ticket.

a. _____
b. _____
c. _____
d. _____

MATCHING REVIEW

Insert the correct word listed in front of each definition below.

appointment book   full-service   retail
business   income   service list
client ticket   inventory   service record
consumption   nails-only
expenses   net worth

17. _____ should include a description of the service, length of time the service takes, and cost of the service
18. _____ supplies used in the business
19. _____ your assets minus your liabilities
20. _____ where the nail technician automatically gets all of the nail care business
21. _____ what you spend
22. _____ list of treatments given and merchandise sold to each client
23. _____ should include client's name, date, service performed, and cost
24. _____ where clients may take nail care more seriously
25. _____ the money you make
26. _____ supplies sold

WORD REVIEW

If you do not know the meanings of the words listed below, look them up in the text.

accountant   income   receipts
advertising   income tax   receptionist
appointment book   independent contractor   rent
benefits   insurance   reputation
booth   inventory   retail supplies
buy   invoices   salary
cancelled checks   laws (local, state, and federal) service record
check stubs   liability   sick days
commission   life insurance   social security
consumption supplies   loss   taxes
daily sales slips   nails-only salon   tips
disability insurance   net worth   tuition
dress code   payroll book   unemployment insurance
employee   personal appointment record   uniform
expenses   petty cash book   ventilation
full-service salon   profit

18

Date _____

Rating _____

Text Pages 228-233

Selling Nail Products and Services

INTRODUCTION

1. List two things nail technicians are responsible for selling.

   a. _____

   b. _____

2. To be successful, the one basic selling goal is
   _____.

3. List five basic steps to selling.

   a. _____

   b. _____

   c. _____

   d. _____

   e. _____

KNOW YOUR PRODUCTS AND SERVICES

4. a. Define feature.
   _____

   b. You learn product features by _____ labels, product bulletins, and industry literature.

   c. What information do you look for on these labels, bulletins, and literature?

      1. _____

      2. _____

      3. _____

      4. _____

5. List five features of nail services.

   a. _____

   b. _____

   c. _____

   d. _____

   e. _____

6. Define benefits.
   _____

7. You will be a good salesperson when you turn the _____ of your products and services into _____ that meet the client's needs and desires.

KNOW WHAT YOUR CLIENT NEEDS AND WANTS

8. When are your client's nail needs discovered or learned?
   _____

9. Explain three questions you will need your client to answer.
   a. _____
   b. _____
   c. _____

10. Two important client lifestyle considerations are
    a. _____
    b. _____

PRESENTING YOUR PRODUCTS AND SERVICES

11. What are two opportunities to sell products and services?
    a. _____
    b. _____

12. While performing a service, tell the client what _____ you are using and why. Suggest that they _____ certain product types and tell them how to use the products. Also discuss other services and the features, _____, and costs of each.

13. List five items that can be included on a service list.
    a. _____
    b. _____
    c. _____
    d. _____
    e. _____

14. While having a service performed, an attractive product display should be in _____ of the client.

15. List five nail maintenance retail products.
    a. _____
    b. _____
    c. _____
    d. _____
    e. _____

ANSWER QUESTIONS AND OBJECTIONS

16. In order to answer client questions, you must be as _____ as possible about your products and services.

17. a. Discuss four items to which a client might object.

    1. _____
    2. _____
    3. _____
    4. _____

    b. You should answer the objection honestly and _____, describing the advantages of the product or service and weighing them against the _____.

CLOSE THE SALE

18. List three steps to closing a sale.

    a. _____
    b. _____
    c. _____

19. What two items should be included on a business card given to the client for their next appointment?

    a. _____
    b. _____

COMPLETION REVIEW

Insert the correct word listed in the sentences below.

appointment	feature	reading
benefit	needs	selling
client consultation	opening a sale	view
closing a sale	products	wearability

21. For success, the one basic selling goal is to meet the _____ of your clients.

22. You learn from product labels, bulletins, and industry literature by _____ them.

23. What a product will do for your client or how it will fulfill your client's needs and wants is a/an _____.

24. Two lifestyle considerations are nail look and _____.

25. Suggestive selling, wrap-up, and scheduling another _____ are three steps to _____.

26. A specific fact about a product or service that describes it is a/an _____.

27. While having a service performed, an attractive product display should be within the client's _____.

28. Your client's nail needs and wants are discovered or learned during the _____.

WORD REVIEW

If you do not know the meanings of the words listed below, look them up in the text.

advantages	lifestyle	salesperson
benefits	maintenance	schedule another appointment
business card	nail look	sell
client consultation	nail problems	service
close the sale	presenting products and services	services
disadvantages	product bulletins	suggested selling
display	products	wearability
features	objections	wrap-up
industry literature	questions	
ingredients	safety precautions	
labels		

Final Review

MULTIPLE CHOICE EXAMINATION

Directions: Read each statement carefully. Choose the best response of the four choices, A, B, C, or D.

1. The thin line of skin at the base of the nail that extends from the nail wall to the nail plate is the
   A. eponychium.
   B. hyponychium.
   C. free edge.
   D. nail groove. _____

2. The type of bacteria that does not produce disease and is often beneficial is
   A. spirilla.
   B. bacilla.
   C. pathogenic.
   D. nonpathogenic. _____

3. John is receiving a pedicure. His toenails should be shaped
   A. straight across.
   B. into a curved shape.
   C. center to corner.
   D. into a pointed shape. _____

4. On a nail tip, the point where the nail plate meets the tip before it is glued to the nail is called the
   A. buffer block.
   B. position stop.
   C. half well.
   D. full well. _____

5. Another name for a kneading massage movement is
   A. effleurage.
   B. friction.
   C. tapotement.
   D. petrissage. _____

119

6. Marion has nail wraps on her nails that are opaque and need colored polish on them. This type of wrap is

   A. linen.

   B. fiberglass.

   C. silk.

   D. None of the above. _____

7. Polish will not stain the nails if the nail technician applies

   A. a top coat.

   B. less than two coats of colored polish.

   C. non-acetone polish remover.

   D. a base coat. _____

8. Tim is studying myology, which is the study of

   A. nerves.

   B. bones.

   C. skin.

   D. muscles. _____

9. Catherine is performing a hand massage on her client Jacquie. The two layers of Jacquie's skin are

   A. papillary and dermis.

   B. papillary and stratum corneum.

   C. dermis and epidermis.

   D. epidermis and stratum corneum. _____

10. The finished acrylic nail on Laura is a/an

    A. monomer.

    B. polymer.

    C. catalyst.

    D. adhesive. _____

11. Mai uses odorless acrylic nails. A difference between odorless and traditional acrylics is that odorless nails

    A. dry faster than traditional acrylics.

    B. can be mixed with any traditional acrylic product.

    C. have no residue when they dry.

    D. are self-leveling. _____

12. Debbie, a salon owner, is adding the money she has spent on equipment, supplies, and uniforms. Debbie is totaling her
    A. profit and loss comparisons.
    B. income.
    C. expenses.
    D. net worth.

13. During a pedicure procedure, the feet are soaked
    A. after the nails are shaped.
    B. at the beginning of the pedicure service.
    C. after the feet are massaged.
    D. immediately before the top coat is applied.

14. An example of a vegetable parasite is
    A. pediculosis.
    B. ringworm.
    C. scabies.
    D. lice.

15. Becca's Nail Salon has installed new ventilation. This ventilation is important for nail technicians and clients because nail products
    A. are flammable.
    B. only come in aerosol sprays.
    C. can cause viral infections.
    D. enter the body through inhalation.

16. Monique's acrylic nails are curing. This means that they are
    A. softening.
    B. weakening.
    C. hardening.
    D. shrinking.

17. The hairlike projections by which bacteria move are called
    A. mitosis.
    B. cocci.
    C. spores.
    D. flagella.

Situation for Items 18-20: *The following four clients have entered your nail salon. Kim, in for a manicure, has white spots on her nail plate. Dick's feet have ringworm, and he would like a pedicure today. Mary has bitten, deformed nails and would like nail tips applied to her natural nails. Peter's nails severely curve over his nail tip/free edge, and he has an appointment for a manicure.*

18. Kim's condition is called
    A. onychauxis.
    B. leukonychia.
    C. onychorrhexis.
    D. agnails. _____

19. Peter's nail condition is called
    A. nail mold.
    B. onychia.
    C. tinea pedis.
    D. onychogryposis. _____

20. The nail technician should refuse to perform a nail service on
    A. Dick.
    B. Kim and Mary.
    C. Dick and Peter.
    D. Mary, Peter, and Kim. _____

21. The nail service where acrylic is added to Karen's new growth area is called
    A. lifting.
    B. rebalancing.
    C. crack repair.
    D. acrylic beads. _____

22. Nails of adults grow at an average of
    A. 1/8 of an inch per week.
    B. 1/8 of an inch per month.
    C. 1/20 of an inch per week.
    D. 1/16 of an inch per month. _____

23. In the matrix are found blood vessels and
    A. lunula.
    B. nerves.
    C. hyponychiums.
    D. cartilage. _____

24. An infected nail should be treated by a
    A. nail technician.
    B. physician.
    C. pharmacist.
    D. cosmetologist. _____

25. In most states, instruments sanitized with hospital-grade disinfectant should be immersed for _____ minutes.
    A. 8
    B. 10
    C. 20
    D. 30 _____

26. The purpose of buffing the nail before applying an acrylic nail is to
    A. remove natural oil.
    B. add color to the nail.
    C. remove acrylic residue.
    D. add gloss to the nail. _____

27. Hangnails are treated by softening the cuticle with
    A. oil.
    B. polish remover.
    C. pumice.
    D. alum. _____

28. The digital bones of the fingers are called
    A. metatarsi.
    B. metacarpi.
    C. phalanges.
    D. clavicles. _____

29. The nevus on Vern's nail was probably caused by:
    A. high blood pressure.
    B. a pigmented mole that occurs in the nail.
    C. poor blood circulation.
    D. the natural immune system. _____

30. Brenda's local beauty supply distributor has given her a Material Data Safety Sheet for the product she uses. This sheet provides information for the product's

    A. instructions on how to apply the product.

    B. chemistry, hazards, and handling procedures.

    C. required sanitation policies and procedures.

    D. percentage of allergic reactions to it. _____

31. Charlotte has a light-cured gel system in her salon. Two light sources for these gels are

    A. ultraviolet and halogen.

    B. ultraviolet and infrared.

    C. infrared and halogen.

    D. visible and infrared. _____

32. The technical term for the nail is

    A. hyponychium.

    B. onyx.

    C. matrix.

    D. cura. _____

33. Ginny's nails will grow faster

    A. in the winter.

    B. as she gets older.

    C. in the summer.

    D. on her feet. _____

34. All of the following statements are true concerning AIDS **EXCEPT** that it

    A. attacks the body's immune system.

    B. is caused by a virus.

    C. lies dormant for many years.

    D. is caused by bacteria. _____

35. Suk is explaining to Cheryl that a particular hand lotion will meet all of Cheryl's needs for her dry hands. Suk, the nail technician, is discussing the hand lotion's

    A. disadvantages.

    B. benefits.

    C. wrap-ups.

    D. features. _____

36. The part of Peggy's nail plate that extends over her fingertips is called the

    A. free edge.

    B. matrix.

    C. hyponychium.

    D. nail bed. _____

37. The ulna is the large bone on the little finger side of the
    A. wrist.
    B. hand.
    C. upper arm
    D. forearm.

38. Before using any manicuring implement, Randy should
    A. wipe it with tissue.
    B. wipe it with a towel.
    C. disinfect it.
    D. wash it with soap and hot water.

39. Melinda is performing a manicure using hot oil and an electric heater. The type of manicure Melinda is performing is
    A. plain water.
    B. French.
    C. reconditioning.
    D. electric.

Situation for Items 40-41: *Kay has a nail problem that was caused when moisture got trapped between her unsanitized natural nails and her artificial nails. This condition was a yellow-green color and has now turned black.*

40. Kay's nail problem is known as
    A. nail mold.
    B. carcinogenic.
    C. rickettsia.
    D. onychophagy.

41. Given Kay's situation, the nail technician should
    A. work on Kay's nails after washing them with an antibacterial soap.
    B. first soak her nails in alcohol for 20 minutes.
    C. first soak her nails in acetone for 20 minutes.
    D. not work on Kay's nails.

42. Juan's wrist bone is called
    A. carpus.
    B. metacarpus.
    C. digit.
    D. radius.

43. Poor-fitting shoes may cause
    A. pterygium.
    B. onychophagy.
    C. ingrown nails.
    D. brittle nails. _____

44. Darryl's hangnails are caused by
    A. a thick lunula.
    B. a thin dermis layer.
    C. an injured matrix.
    D. dry cuticles. _____

45. The type of polish remover to use on clients who have artificial nails is
    A. acetone.
    B. non-acetone.
    C. alcohol.
    D. hydrogen peroxide. _____

46. The radial artery supplies the
    A. thumb side of the arm.
    B. little finger side of the arm.
    C. palm of the hand.
    D. back of the hand. _____

47. While performing a pedicure, Anita should use _____ to separate her client's toes.
    A. paper towels
    B. her fingers
    C. toe separators
    D. her orangewood stick _____

48. When using quarternary ammonium compound, one important step is to
    A. measure it carefully.
    B. change it after each use.
    C. change it daily.
    D. dilute it to an antiseptic strength. _____

49. The nail technician should file Tony's fingernails
    A. from center to each corner.
    B. from each corner to the center.
    C. straight across.
    D. back and forth. _____

50. Mai uses quats to disinfect her implements. Another name for quats is
    A. sodium hypochlorite compound.
    B. formaldehyde.
    C. quaternary ammonium compound.
    D. ethyl alcohol. _____

51. Mark is applying a form of nail art that uses very fragile leafing. This type of nail art is
    A. gems
    B. striping tape.
    C. foil.
    D. air-brushing. _____

52. Tinea pedis is another name for
    A. hangnails.
    B. ingrown nails.
    C. athlete's foot.
    D. brittle nails. _____

53. The ulnar nerve supplies the
    A. thumb side of the arm.
    B. little finger side of the arm.
    C. fingers.
    D. wrist. _____

54. The deep fold of skin in which Mary's nail root is lodged is called the
    A. nail fold or mantle.
    B. nail groove.
    C. eponychium.
    D. lunula. _____

55. It is important to sanitize a client's nails before applying acrylic nails because the antiseptic will
    A. adhere or attach the acrylic to the natural nail.
    B. soften the nail properly for acrylics.
    C. help prevent fungus from forming.
    D. dry the acrylic quickly. _____

56. Korbi is placing his manicuring implements in a disinfectant solution. The type of sanitizer he is using is a/an
    A. ultraviolet sanitizer.
    B. disinfection container.
    C. autoclave.
    D. dry sanitizer. _____

57. The name of Tom's skin coloring pigment is
    A. lymph.
    B. keratin.
    C. sebum.
    D. melanin. _____

58. The parts of a muscle are
    A. origin, digits, and belly.
    B. origin, insertion, and belly.
    C. digits, insertion, and phalanges.
    D. insertion, belly, and phalanges. _____

59. Sara, a nail technician, should apply nail polish in strokes that are
    A. rough and jerky.
    B. quick and smooth.
    C. short and dry.
    D. long and excessively wet. _____

60. Emil should store his dirty/soiled towels in _____ until he has time to launder them.
    A. a bin at the shampoo area
    B. an open container for soiled items
    C. a closed container for soiled items
    D. the manicuring drawer _____

61. What does a disinfectant do to bacteria? It
    A. kills all bacteria.
    B. kills only pathogenic bacteria.
    C. retards bacteria growth.
    D. retards only pathogenic bacteria growth. _____

62. Ron, a nail technician, has just completed a manicure and is cleaning up his table area. Ron is to discard all of the following used items EXCEPT the
    A. cuticle nippers.
    B. emery board.
    C. orangewood stick.
    D. cotton balls. _____

63. The nail plate is made up of a protein called
    A. collagen.
    B. melanin.
    C. keratin.
    D. sebum.

64. Maria's rubber implements should not be disinfected with
    A. phenolics.
    B. quaternary ammonium compound.
    C. sodium hypochlorite compound.
    D. fumigant tablets.

65. Nail technicians use nail forms when they apply
    A. nail tips.
    B. acrylic nails.
    C. mending tissue.
    D. acrylic over nail tips.

66. The nail plate, or body, extends from the nail root to the
    A. lunula.
    B. matrix.
    C. nail bed.
    D. free edge.

67. While nipping her client's cuticles, Lisa accidentally cuts into the skin, and it begins to bleed. Lisa should apply to the cut
    A. alum.
    B. disinfectant.
    C. 70% ethyl alcohol.
    D. a styptic pencil.

68. Lee's sudoriferous glands
    A. regulate his body temperature.
    B. are commonly known as oil glands.
    C. empty into his hair follicles.
    D. secrete sebum.

69. In some states, formalin
    A. cannot be used.
    B. is felt to be the safest disinfectant.
    C. is used to sanitize hands.
    D. must be FDA registered.

70. The nail grooves are indentations found at the _____ of the nail.

   A. base

   B. sides

   C. root

   D. free edge _____

71. The maintenance of the normal, internal stability of Ellen's body is known as

   A. homeostasis.

   B. leukonychia.

   C. carcinogenic.

   D. onychogryposis. _____

72. Carlos is putting an antiseptic on his client's nails in preparation for artificial nails. An antiseptic

   A. kills only pathogenic bacteria.

   B. kills only nonpathogenic bacteria.

   C. kills all bacteria.

   D. slows bacteria growth. _____

73. Sandy is preparing her client's natural nails for acrylics. Which of the following must Sandy do to the natural nail(s) before applying the acrylic?

   A. soften it with cream

   B. buff it to remove the shine

   C. soak it in hot oil

   D. soak for 10 minutes in warm soapy water _____

74. Sue hears, smells, tastes, touches, and sees well. Her five senses are under the control of her _____ nervous system.

   A. peripheral

   B. neurological

   C. central

   D. autonomic _____

75. Nails by Natalie, The Nail Clinic, and Bertha's Beauty Salon all use the same disinfection method. The most common method that salons use is _____ disinfection.

   A. physical

   B. steam or moist heat

   C. chemical

   D. autoclave _____

SCORING

Number of Items Wrong:	Score:*
0	100%
1	99%
2	97%
3	96%
4	95%
5	93%
6	92%
7	91%
8	89%
9	88%
10	87%
11	85%
12	84%
13	83%
14	81%
15	80%
16	79%
17	77%
18	76%
19 or more	fail

* = There are 75 items on this test. Each item is worth 1.33 points. Because of this, some percentages in the score column are missed, or the score column does not list every percentage chronogically.